Incredible Edibles

by Eriann Hullquist

Third Edition

TEACH Services, Inc.
Brushton, New York

PRINTED IN CANADA

World rights reserved. This book or any portion thereof may not be copied or reproduced in any form or manner whatever, except as provided by law, without the written permission of the publisher, except by a reviewer who may quote brief passages in a review.

1999 00 01 02 03 04 05 06 07 08 · 5 4 3 2 1

The author assumes full responsibility for the accuracy of all facts and quotations as cited in this book.

Copyright © 1999 TEACH Services, Inc.

ISBN 1-57258-135-2
Library of Congress Catalog Card No. 98-84773

Published by

TEACH Services, Inc.
254 Donovan road
Brushton, New York 12916

Acknowledgments

A special thanks to my good friends, Pat and Doug McCarthy, owners of The Harrisville Squires Inn, Harrisville, New Hampshire, who so graciously gave of their time, talents and environment to create the settings for the color photos. I also want to thank to Mark Corliss, owner of Multi-Media Creations in Keene, New Hampshire whose patience was so appreciated as his expertise was utilized setting up each photo, to achieve just the right effect.

Dedication

To my husband Timothy, whose candid remarks and suggestions motivated me to continue on to get the right taste and texture. Also, to our three children Sarah, Phillip and Janelle, who both consented and dissented to try my newest creations.

Dear Friend,

My first exposure to the concept of being a total vegetarian (vegan) held visions of eating carrot sticks and alfalfa sprouts for the rest of my life; that did not hold my attention long! It took working at a health institute to see the health results of this diet and then many years of experimenting to develop these recipes.

The recipes I have included in this cookbook are part of a monthly meal planner. It is my desire that they will tantalize your tastebuds and convince you that eating a plant-based diet can be very satisfying.

At the time of this writing, I am a wife and mother of three teenage children. We all work in the family business and do homeschool; so that does not leave us a whole lot of time to spend in the kitchen. Therefore, these recipes do not consume a lot of time, and I have also chosen them for their ease of preparation, even if you are a novice to vegan cooking. The ingredients are user friendly and those few items that are not available in a regular grocery store, you can substitute easily if you choose.

I have written personal notes alongside of each recipe, so I could be with you while you use this cookbook.

Have a great time and "cherish each bite!"

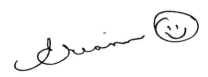

Timothy's Testimony

Before I married Eriann, I ate the majority of my meals in restaurants. By contrast, she had been immersed in a culture of preventive health that had a major emphasis of not eating anything that could not be digested easily within 5–6 hours. Our eating habits and tastes clashed tremendously.

However, now I would much rather eat at home; and I am delighted to invite friends and clients home for a meal. We enjoy an abundance and variety that I feel is far superior to anything that I have had in the past. And those items that I have given up have been replaced by something better.

I would like to interest you in this book because I know you will experience delightful meals while enjoying an increase in your quality of life.

— Timothy Hullquist

CONTENTS

- INGREDIENTS LIST 8
- WEEKLY HEALTH PLANNER 10
- "GARDENS" PRINCIPLES. 10
- MONTHLY MEAL PLANNER 11
- MONTHLY MEAL PLANNER 12
- FRUIT RECIPES 13
- VEGETABLE RECIPES 37
- GRAINS RECIPES. 63
  - COOKING GRAINS CHART 63
- BEAN RECIPES. 85
  - COOKING BEANS CHART. 85
- NUTS & SEEDS RECIPES 101
- MISCELLANEOUS. 113
- KID'S KORNER 131
- INDEX 141

INGREDIENTS LIST

Here is a list of all the ingredients used in this book.

FRESH	Fruits:	apples, bananas, berries, oranges, peaches, rhubarb
	Vegetables:	beets, carrots, onions, potatoes, turnips, garlic cloves, green onions, iceberg lettuce, chicory, spinach, romaine, endive, parsley, alfalfa sprouts, kale, cabbage, cucumbers, eggplant, green peppers, tomatoes, winter squash, yellow crookneck squash, zucchini, broccoli, cabbage (red & green), cauliflower, celery
FROZEN	Concentrates:	apple, grape, orange, pineapple, white grape, white grape-peach, white grape-raspberry
	Other:	bananas, berries, blueberries, strawberries
DRIED	Fruit:	apples, apricots, dates, prunes, raisins
	Other:	garbanzos, navy beans, soy beans, pinto beans, onions, lentils, split peas
CANNED	Fruits:	applesauce, cranberry sauce, crushed pineapple, peaches, pineapple juice, coconut milk
	Vegetables:	black olives, green chilies, sweet pickle relish, tomato juice, tomato paste, tomato sauce, water chestnuts, whole kernel corn, green beans, chopped tomatoes, kidney beans
GRAINS/FLOURS		whole wheat flour, unbleached white flour, soy flour, oats (regular & quick) gluten flour, whole wheat pastry flour, long grain brown rice, rye flour, wheatgerm, bulgur wheat, couscous, whole grain cornmeal, millet
SEEDS/NUTS		raw and roasted cashews, shredded coconut, sunflower seeds, sesame seeds, flax seeds, walnuts, pecans
SWEETENERS		barley malt, carob chips, corn syrup, honey, maple syrup, molasses, Sucanat®
FLAVORINGS	Sweet:	orange peel, lemon peel, coriander, cardamon, vanilla, maple extract, lemon extract
	Savory:	sage, parsley flakes, sweet basil, paprika, cumin, oregano, garlic powder, thyme, chives, onion powder, lemon juice, celery salt, cilantro
	Other:	taco seasoning, chicken-style seasoning, nutritional yeast flakes, Bragg's Liquid Aminos, carob powder, salt, Italian seasoning
MISCELLANEOUS		ENER-G Foods baking powder, TVP, vegeburger, Emes gelatin, Minute Tapioca, baking yeast, cornstarch, vegetable oil, olive oil, dairy-free milk, silken tofu, bacon-like bits, corn tortillas, Soya Kaas mozzarella cheese, assorted pasta

HELPFUL HINTS

Recipes:

1. Always read the whole recipe FIRST.
2. Each recipe calls attention to a specific food item, which is in bold.
3. Each recipe is a quantity to feed 4–6 people.
4. Each recipe has been calculated to have the minimal amount of steps possible.

Substitutions:

What you can use if you do not have:

Bragg's Liquid Aminos = soy sauce

ENER-G Foods Baking Powder = use ½ the amount of regular baking powder

Emes Gelatin = regular gelatin

Sucanat® = brown sugar

Dairy-free milk = regular milk

Equipment:

1. My blender is my best friend (but not all blenders are created equal)— Some are stronger and some have a larger capacity.
2. Temperatures of ovens can vary; check frequently the first time baking a recipe.

Ingredients:

1. Always use fresh ingredients. It does make a difference in the taste of the finished product.
2. Measure seasonings accurately; with whole foods you can throw in a little extra and it will not matter, but seasonings are a different matter.
3. Whole wheat flour and unbleached white flour each give a different texture... experiment!

WEEKLY HEALTH PLANNER

Activity	Portion	Time	Sun.	Mon.	Tues.	Wed.	Thurs.	Fri.	Sat.
Sleep		7–8 hours							
Water	2 cups	5 min.							
Fresh Fruit	**2 pieces**	**15 min.**							
Grain Cereal	**1 cup**	**15 min.**							
Water	2 cups	5 min.							
Sunbath		10 min.							
No Eating Between									
Fresh Vegetable Salad	**2 cups**	**15 min.**							
Meal Portions		**15 min.**							
Water	2 cups	5 min.							
Walk 2+ miles		30 min.							
Water	2 cups	5 min.							
No Eating Between									
Popcorn/Zwieback									
Melons									
Video View									

"GARDENS" PRINCIPLES

God's Love	"Why do you spend money for what is not bread, and your wages for what does not satisfy? Listen carefully to Me, and eat what is good, and let your soul delight itself in abundance." *Isaiah 55:2*
Air	Breathe deeply while exercising.
Rest	Get a minimum of 7 hours of sleep per night. (the hours you sleep before 12 midnight are worth 2 hours of sleep gotten after midnight).
Diet	(A) Eat fresh food first. It is **THE** most important food you will eat all day! (B) Allow 5–6 hours between meals (from the beginning of one meal to the beginning of the next meal). (C) Do not eat ANYTHING between meals. (D) Allow a minimum of 30 minutes to eat and no longer than 60 minutes to finish the last bite. (E) Chew each bite of food so it is thoroughly mixed with saliva.
Exercise	Walk briskly (non-stop) for 30 minutes outdoors. Negative ions make for positive thoughts!. There is no "bad" weather; only "bad" clothing. The goal is a minimum of 2 miles in this time period.
No Abuse	No alcohol, coffee, tea, colas or tobacco in any form.
Sunshine	Take a 10 minute sunbath each day. This could be part of your walk.

MONTHLY MEAL PLANNER

BREAKFAST

Breads	Baked Dishes	Pie	Savory	Cereal	Dessert	Fruit Over Grain
Blueberry Breakfast Cake	Rhubarb Crisp	Mud	Scrambled Tofu	Delicious Millet	Tofu Cheesecake	French Toast
Sweet Rolls	Cranapple Bake	Coconut Cream	Hash Browns	Spiced Rice	Butterscotch Pudding	Waffles
Banana Nut Bread	Prune Crisp	Blueberry	Chip Beef Gravy Biscuits	Granola Strawberry Yogurt	Carob Prune Cake	Pancakes
Breakfast Muffins	Berry Good Cobbler	Pumpkin	Tofu Omelet	Lemon Chiffon Cornmeal	Strawberry Shortcake	Applesauce Toast

LUNCH

Casserole	Bean Dishes	Pasta	Vegetable Soup	Bean Soup	Fast Foods	Mexican
Cabbage Rolls Fried Rice	Birdseed Bread Black Beans	Stroganoff Rice	Cream of Potato Chicken Salad	Navy Bean Tabouli	Vegeburgers Ketchup	Mexican Soup
Pecan Roast Scalloped Potatoes	Chili Cornbread	Macaroni & Cheese Chunky Green Salad	Borsch 3 Bean Salad	Split Pea Soup Pasta Salad	Pizza Chick Pea Salad	Enchiladas
Stuffed Peppers Glazed Beets	Sweet Beans Potato Salad	Lasagna Chlorophyll Salad	Tomato Soup Reubens	"Chicken" Rice Winter Squash	Meal in a Peel Sunshine Loaf	Burritos Salsa
Cheez Potatoes Coleslaw	Savory Soybeans Eggplant–Zucchini	Spaghetti & Meatballs	Minestrone Eggless Salad	Esau's Pottage Tamale Pie	Sloppy Joes Summer Garden Salad	Tacos Salsa

SUPPER OPTIONS and DESSERTS

Drink	Cold Fruit Dish	Hot Fruit Dish	Fresh Fruit	Grain	Cookies	Cookies
Orange Julius	Orange Ambrosia	Fruit Soup	Honeydew	Zwieback	Coconut Macaroons	Seed Samplers
Banana Fruit Shake	Pineapple Pudding	Apricot Couscous	Cantaloupe	Popcorn	Maple Pecan Cookies	Bird's Nest
Cup of Carob	Tropical Fruit Gel	Baked Apple	Watermelon	Rice Cake	Nut Butter Cookies	Date Nut Chews

INCREDIBLE EDIBLES

MONTHLY MEAL PLANNER

BREAKFAST

Breads	Baked Dishes	Pie	Savory	Cereal	Dessert	Fruit Over Grain

LUNCH

Casserole	Bean Dishes	Pasta	Vegetable Soup	Bean Soup	Fast Foods	Mexican

SUPPER OPTIONS AND DESSERTS

Drink	Cold Fruit Dish	Hot Fruit Dish	Fresh Fruit	Grain	Cookies	Cookies

FRUIT RECIPES

Definition: The class of foods that are grown on vines, bushes and trees. They are preceded by a flower and you can visibly see the seed(s) in or on it.

This is what I routinely have on hand (or that is in season):

Fresh– apples, bananas, cantaloupe, grapefruit, grapes, kiwi, oranges, peaches, pears, plums.

Canned– applesauce, apricots, cherries, crushed pineapple, pineapple juice, peaches, pears, lemon juice.

Dried– apples, apricots, bananas, dates, figs, prunes, raisins.

Frozen– apple concentrate, bananas, blueberries, orange concentrate, pineapple concentrate, raspberries, strawberries, white grape juice concentrate.

Banana Fruit Shake

2 cups bite-size pieces of frozen **banana**
2 cups [approximately] pineapple juice
2 cups [approximately] partially thawed, frozen strawberries

In a blender, put frozen bananas, and barely cover with pineapple juice. Turn blender on and add strawberries one at a time until it will not blend anymore (use a rubber spatula to scrape down the sides as it is blending). Serve immediately.

This has got to be one of our all-time summer favorites. When my nephew asked for 'seconds' (he eats almost exclusively at fast-food restaurants), I knew it was a hit.

Banana Nut Bread

⅔	cup very warm water
2	Tbsp. baking yeast
⅔	cup honey
⅓	cup maple syrup
½	cup vegetable oil
2	tsp. each: salt and vanilla
2–3	mashed ripe **bananas**
1	cup pecans or walnuts, chopped
3	cups whole wheat/unbleached white

In a 2 cup measuring cup put water and yeast and set aside for 10–15 minutes (or until bubbled up).

In a medium mixing bowl, put honey, maple syrup, oil, salt, vanilla, and bananas; cream with a mixer for 3–6 minutes. Add nuts, yeast mixture, flour, and mix well by hand. Put in small loaf pans ⅔ full and let rise for 60 minutes. Then carefully (so you do not make the yeast 'fall') bake in 325° oven for approximately 20–30 minutes.

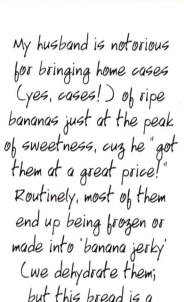

My husband is notorious for bringing home cases (yes, cases!) of ripe bananas just at the peak of sweetness, cuz he "got them at a great price!" Routinely, most of them end up being frozen or made into 'banana jerky' (we dehydrate them; but this bread is a delightful 'home' for some of them.

PINEAPPLE PUDDING

2	cups **pineapple** juice
¾	cup coconut milk
½	cup shredded coconut
¼	cup each: cornstarch and honey
1	tsp. vanilla
¼	tsp. salt
1	can [15 oz.] crushed **pineapple**, with juice

In a blender, blend all ingredients except crushed pineapple. Remove to a saucepan, add crushed pineapple and cook this mixture over medium high heat, stirring constantly until thickened. Pour into serving dish and chill.

This pudding is a refreshing summer breakfast fare... makes one think of coconut palms, pineapple plantations, sun and ocean breezes... ahhh!

Whole Grain Waffles (p.79) topped with Strawberries and Sweet Cream ➤

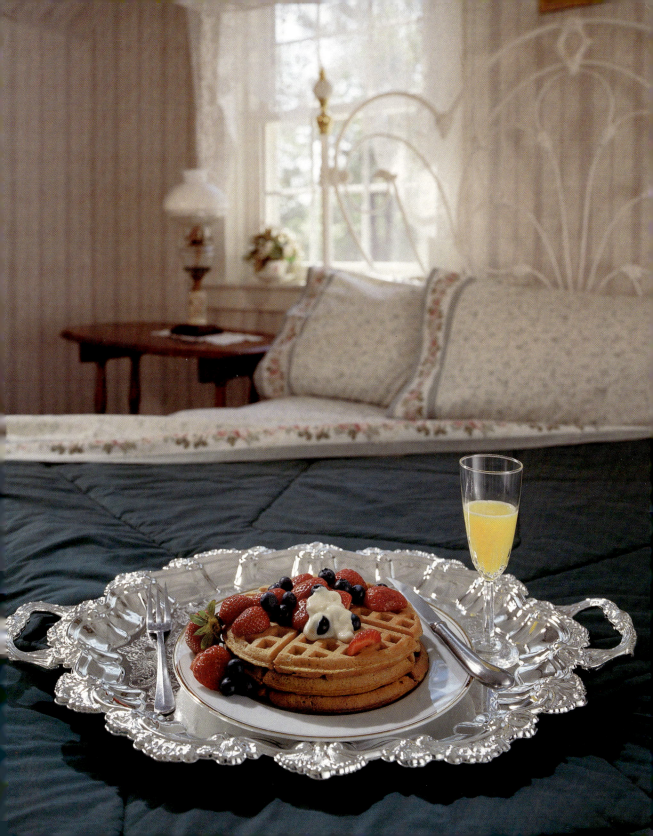

Lemon Chiffon Pudding

½	cup whole grain yellow cornmeal
1	cup cold water/dairy-free milk
1	cup raw cashew pieces
1	cup boiling water
¾	cup honey
½	cup **lemon juice**
2	Tbsp. Emes gelatin
1	tsp. each: lemon peel and vanilla
½	tsp. each: salt and lemon extract

In a saucepan, mix cornmeal and cold water. Then cook over medium heat and stir constantly until it thickens to paste consistency. Remove from heat.

In a blender, blend cashews and boiling water until smooth. Add the cornmeal mixture and all the rest of the ingredients and blend until totally mixed and completely smooth (about 2–3 minutes). Pour into serving dish and chill in refrigerator until firm (about 2–3 hours).

This pudding is delicious. I first tasted it at a small college cafeteria and was so surprised to find out that the basic ingredients were cornmeal and cashews. I think you will be pleasantly surprised also.

Carob Prune Cake

1	cup pitted **prunes**, diced
1¼	cup boiling water
½	cup each Sucanat® and honey
⅓	vegetable oil
1	tsp. vanilla

1	cup whole wheat pastry flour
1	cup unbleached white flour
2	Tbsp. carob powder
1	Tbsp. ENER-G Foods baking powder
1	tsp. each: coriander and cardamon
½	tsp. salt

In a mixing bowl, mix the first section (wet ingredients). In a mixing bowl, mix second section (dry ingredients). Add wet mixture to dry mixture and mix until most lumps have disappeared. Spoon into greased cake pan and immediately bake in 325° oven for approximately 35–40 minutes (or until toothpick inserted in center comes out clean). Frost with coconut cream frosting.

My Dad put himself through school in S. California working in the bakery. Having some extra stewed prunes lying around, he added them (instead of the applesauce) to the chocolate cake he was making—it was a tremendous success. This is our vegan carob version.

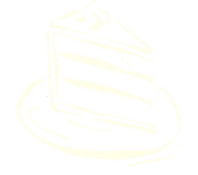

Prune Crisp

2	cups pitted **prunes**
1	cup dried apples (or other kind)
1	can [12 oz.] thawed apple juice concentrate
1	can [12 oz.] water
2	cups raw wheat germ
2	cups quick oats
½	tsp. salt
⅓	cup vegetable oil
⅓	cup fruit juice (any kind)

Put prunes and dried apples through a food chopper (or cut up by hand) so they are in very small pieces.

In a saucepan, put prunes, apples, water and apple juice concentrate and heat up until all is very hot. Remove from heat.

In a mixing bowl, mix wheatgerm, rolled oats, and salt together. Then mix in oil and fruit juice until the mixture is crumbly. Spread ½ of this crumb mixture in the bottom of a casserole dish. Spread all of the prune mixture over this and top with the remaining crumb mixture. Bake in 325° oven for 35 minutes. Serve warm.

This was voted the most favorite breakfast dish at a cooking school. The key to the success of this recipe is to make sure your prunes taste good to start with and are not too dry.

Strawberry Shortcake

2	cups whole **strawberries**
1	can [12 oz.] white grape juice concentrate
2	Tbsp. cornstarch
2	cups of cut up **strawberries**

In a blender, blend whole strawberries. In a saucepan mix white grape juice concentrate with cornstarch. Stir and cook over medium high heat until thickened; then add cut up strawberries and blended strawberries and mix all together. Serve warm over biscuits.

Do the words 'strawberry shortcake' make your mouth water? Use this sauce over warm biscuits, top with a scoop of sweet cream and you'll enjoy our home-style version. It is ummmmm good!! (Also great over waffles!)

Strawberry Yogurt

1	cup boiling water
¾	cup raw cashew pieces

2	cups pineapple juice
⅓	cup each: honey and cornstarch
¼	tsp. salt

3–4	cups **strawberries** (frozen or fresh)

In a blender, blend water and cashews; add all the rest of the ingredients and blend until smooth. Pour into a saucepan and cook over medium heat, stirring constantly until thickened. Transfer to serving bowl and refrigerate.

My friend, Christin, shared the basics for this recipe as one that is 'out of this world.' I'm not naturally a yogurt lover, but this is a delightful breakfast-type dish topped with granola.

Blueberry Breakfast Cake

A great way to enjoy blueberries in the winter... hot right out of the oven!

2	cups bread flour (combination whole wheat pastry and unbleached white)
¼	cup rye flour
1	Tbsp. ENER-G Foods baking powder
1	tsp. salt
1	cup dairy-free milk
¼	cup each: honey and applesauce
2	Tbsp. vegetable oil
1	tsp. vanilla
1	cup **blueberries**, frozen or fresh

In a mixing bowl, mix the first section (dry ingredients). Add second section (wet ingredients) and mix just enough to moisten and without lumps. Fold in blueberries. Spoon into shallow casserole dish and bake in 325° oven for 30 minutes (or longer if necessary).

Note to make like a coffee cake, drizzle maple syrup across the top and sprinkle Sucanat® BEFORE baking. Also, I use an 8x8 size casserole dish to bake it in.

Blueberry Pie

- 1 can [12 oz.] white grape juice concentrate
- ½ can [12 oz.] water
- 4 Tbsp. each: cornstarch, Sucanat® and Minute Tapioca

- 1 can [15 oz.] crushed pineapple
- 4 cups [16 oz. pkg.] **blueberries**

In a saucepan, mix white grape juice concentrate, water, cornstarch, Sucanat® and Minute Tapioca. Let set for 10–15 minutes. Add blueberries and crushed pineapple. Heat up over medium high heat, stirring frequently until thickened. Spoon into crust and bake in 325° oven for 30–40 minutes.

Note: it will all turn blue once it is hot and thickened.

In the summer, our trek up Gap Mountain, NH, puts us in the midst of blueberries for miles. What a 'feast of fresh' we have at lunchtime! Once our five gallon bucket is full we lug it back home to wind up in pies.

Apricot Jam

dried **apricots**
pineapple juice

Fill a saucepan ½ full of dried apricots (we like Turkish the best) and cover with pineapple juice. Let this set for several hours or overnight. Then heat the mixture until it is very hot, stirring frequently to make sure that it does not burn. Spoon approximately 2 cups at a time of this mixture into the blender and blend until perfectly smooth (add additional pineapple juice as needed). Spoon, scrape or pour into pint or quart canning jars. Refrigerate.

Note: You can process these in a water bath according to canning directions, if you plan on making a large batch.

This jam is more correctly called 'Daddy's Jam' in our home. It always has been (and probably always will be) his all-time favorite. He parts with a pint each year as a gift to his 'birthday buddy,' Laurie.

Apricot Couscous

8	dried **apricots**, cut up small
1	cup coconut milk (or any dairy-free milk)
1	cup water
1	tsp. vegetable oil
1	squirt of honey from the honey bear
¼	tsp. each: salt and cardamon

1	cup couscous

In a saucepan, bring to a boil all the ingredients in the first section. Remove from heat and stir in couscous; cover and let set for 5 minutes or until all the liquid is absorbed. Fluff with a fork and serve immediately.

Note: If you wait too long before you fluff it with a fork, it will congeal and then you will have to slice it to serve! Also, we like the Turkish apricots the best.

This is one of the quickest, yummiest dishes when time is at a premium.

Fruit Soup

3	cups **pineapple** juice
2	cups water
½	cup Minute Tapioca
2	cups dried fruit **(apples, apricots, prunes, raisins)**
2	cups canned fruit **(peaches, pears, pineapple)**
4	**bananas** (optional)

In a saucepan, mix the pineapple juice, water and tapioca. Set aside for 10 minutes. Cut up all dried fruit in small pieces and cut up canned fruit, (if necessary). Put all fruit into the saucepan and bring to a boil (stirring frequently to prevent scorching). Lower heat to simmer and cook until tapioca is clear.

Note: you may need to add more water or juice to get the consistency you want.

A delightful soup eaten with muffins on a cold, wintry day! This is a recipe that will always be a favorite for those of us who live in the north country amid snow and ice. It warms the insides and tastes fantastic.

Fruit/Nut Bites

1 cup each: dried **apricots**, pitted **dates**, **raisins**, and **walnuts**

equal parts of honey & orange juice concentrate

shredded coconut

Put each of the dried fruits through a food chopper on the coarse setting. Remove to a mixing bowl and add a spoonful at a time of the honey and orange concentrate mixture until the dried fruit/nut mixture holds together. Form walnut-size balls and roll in shredded coconut. Refrigerate.

These treats are a fun edible gift to give at Christmas time. They are truly a 'little bite of goodness.'

Orange Ambrosia

1	can [12 oz.] **orange** juice concentrate
3	cans [12 oz.] water
½	cup shredded coconut
½	cup Minute Tapioca
¼	cup honey
3	fresh **oranges**, peeled

In a saucepan, mix everything (except fresh orange). Set this aside for 10–15 minutes.

Cut up the oranges into bite-size pieces. After the 10 minutes is up, stir the orange juice mixture over medium high heat until thickened. Remove from the heat and fold in the fresh oranges. Spoon into a serving dish and refrigerate. Serve chilled.

Our daughter Janelle especially loves to visit my sister's southern California home where citrus is in abundance. She gets to eat all she wants of this sunny gold without restraint of quantity or price!

Orange Julius

1	whole **orange**, peeled
½	can [12 oz.] **orange** juice concentrate
⅓	cup dairy-free milk powder
¼	cup honey
½	tsp. **orange** peel
2	cups ice
	OR…
1½	cups dairy-free milk and 6–8 ice cubes
	water enough to blend

In a blender, blend all of the ingredients. Serve immediately.

Note: only add additional water if necessary to make blender blend.

This is actually our son Phillip's rendition of a mall favorite. Try it and see if you like it!

Cranapple Bake

6	cups **apples** peeled, cored and shredded
1	can [16 oz.] jellied **cranberry** sauce
1	cup quick oats
½	cup whole wheat flour
½	cup chopped walnuts
⅓	cup Sucanat®
¼	cup vegetable oil
½	tsp. cardamon
¼	tsp. salt

In a mixing bowl, mix apples and cranberry sauce together. Put in a casserole dish. In the bowl, put all the rest of the ingredients and mix together. Spoon over the apple-cranberry mixture. Bake in 325° oven for 30–40 minutes.

Note: you can use jellied OR whole berry sauce.

I used to live in the midst of acres of cranberry bogs and could have all I wanted. What to do with it? This fruit looks so colorful when cooked up; but as my roommate found out very quickly, one needs to add SOMETHING to it to make it palatable!

Cranberry Relish

2	cups fresh **cranberries**, chopped
1	fresh hard firm red apple, shredded
1	fresh orange, cut up in little pieces
½	cup walnuts, chopped fine
	honey to sweeten

In a mixing bowl, mix all ingredients together. Chill before serving.

I asked my friend Mary from church to make a fresh cranberry relish for one of our holiday dinners. This is what she came up with, and we all loved it. I had to get her to put down some kind of quantities cuz she comes from the era of 'handful of this, dash of that, and a bit of this!'

Berry Good Cobbler

1	cup whole wheat flour
1	cup Sucanat®
2	Tbsp. ENER-G Foods baking powder
¼	tsp. salt
1	cup dairy-free milk
¼	cup vegetable oil
4–6	cups fresh **berries** (any kind)

In a mixing bowl, mix first section (dry ingredients) and then add the second section (wet ingredients). Pour into baking dish and spoon the berries into the middle. Bake in 325° oven for approximately 30 minutes.

Note: although blackberries, raspberries and blueberries are usually first choice, fresh sliced peaches taste good also.

My cousin Cindy got me onto this recipe. I was visiting her one summer and was enthralled with the blackberries strewn all over their property out back. I picked to my heart's content for 60 minutes or so, and she put together this cobbler in about 5 minutes! It was so berry good! I think you'll agree.

Sweet Rolls (p.74) are cause for celebration—a veritable favorite! ➤

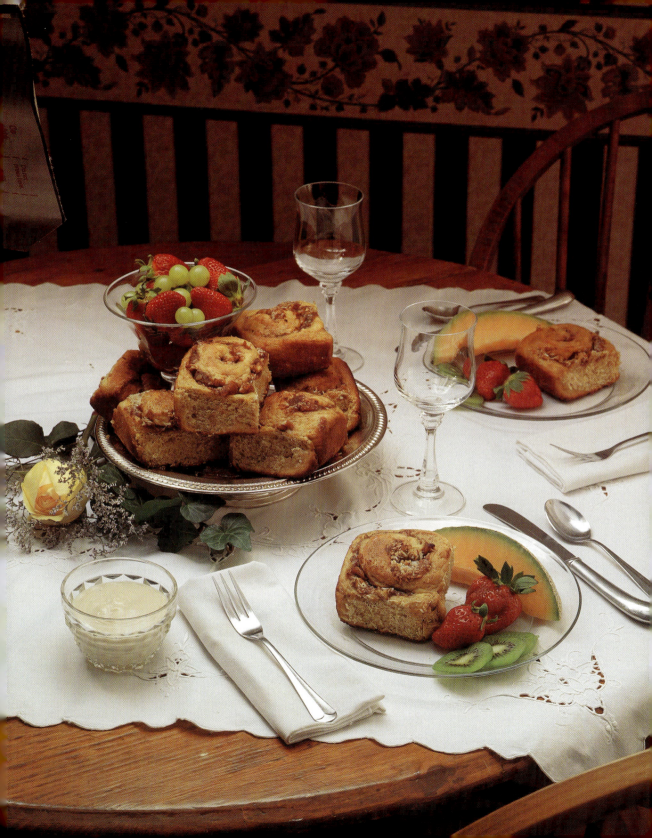

Rhubarb Crisp

6	cups fresh **rhubarb**, diced
1	cup Sucanat®
1	can [12 oz.] white grape juice concentrate
3	Tbsp. Minute Tapioca
1	Tbsp. orange peel
1	tsp. lemon peel
3	cups bread crumbs
⅓	cup vegetable oil
1	tsp. vanilla
¼	tsp. salt

In a saucepan mix the first section (first six ingredients) together and set aside for 10 minutes. Then cook over medium heat until it is soft.

In a mixing bowl, mix second section (last four ingredients) together. In a casserole dish layer rhubarb and crumb mixture alternately. Bake in 325° oven for 40 minutes. Serve hot with a cream of your choice.

We have loads of rhubarb in the early spring. What to do with this VERY tart water-laden produce?? This is one wonderful way...!!

Tropical Fruit Gel

1   cup boiling water

3   Tbsp. Emes gelatin

1   can [12 oz.] white grape raspberry concentrate (or any kind that's colorful)

1   can [12 oz.] water

2   cups canned fruit, drained & cut in small pieces
(peaches, pears, pineapple)

In a mixing bowl, stir water and gelatin powder until dissolved. Add concentrate and water. Pour into dish, add fruit and refrigerate until jelled.

The kids had this gel at a camp supper, and it was a hit with everyone.

Peach Crisp

¼	cup cornstarch
¼	cup cold water
1	can [12 oz.] white grape peach concentrate
1	can [12 oz.] water
1	Tbsp. lemon juice
8	cups canned peaches, sliced/diced
	granola

In a saucepan, mix cornstarch and water. Add white grape peach concentrate, water and lemon juice. Over medium high heat, cook until thickened, stirring constantly. Add peaches, mix together and pour into casserole dish; top with granola. Cover with foil and bake in 325° oven for 30–40 minutes.

This is the crisp I make up if I am really pressed for time. Granola is our standby when all else fails and is a great substitute for getting out all the crisp topping ingredients.

Applesauce Toast

whole wheat bread

nut butter
(peanut butter, almond or cashew)

applesauce

berries

granola

I think the kids would enjoy this breakfast at least every other day if that's what was served. Very fast! Very good!

Toast the bread; add enough berries (of any kind) to the applesauce to make it colorful. Heat it up on the stove or in the microwave. Spread nut butter on toast, place on plate and spoon hot applesauce over it and sprinkle granola on top. Eat it as you would French toast.

VEGETABLE RECIPES

Definition: The edible portions of the plant.

This is what I routinely keep on hand from the garden (frozen, canned, or root cellar) or buy when the price is right.

Root *– beets, carrots, onions, potatoes, radishes, sweet potatoes, turnips.*

Leaf *– beet greens, cabbage, kale, lettuce, spinach, swiss chard.*

Stem *– asparagus, celery.*

Flower *– broccoli, brussels sprouts, cauliflower.*

Fruit/Vegetables *– summer squash, winter squash, green peppers, snapbeans, tomatoes, cucumbers, zucchini.*

BEST METHODS FOR COOKING VEGETABLES

1. *Cook in smallest amount of water; add vegetables after water has already started to boil.*
2. *Cook as short a time as possible.*
3. *Avoid soaking vegetables.*
4. *Keep vegetables cold until ready to cook.*
5. *Avoid the use of utensils that have copper alloys or are made of aluminum.*
6. *Use a stiff brush for cleaning vegetables.*
7. *Cook vegetables whole or in large pieces when possible. Cook with skins on to save nutrients.*
8. *Serve as soon as possible after vegetable is cooked.*

KETCHUP

1	can [15 oz.] **tomato** sauce
1	can [6 oz.] **tomato** paste
½	cup each: Sucanat® and lemon juice
1	Tbsp. onion powder
1	tsp. each: paprika, salt, sweet basil
½	tsp. each: cumin, oregano, garlic powder

In a blender, blend all ingredients together until very smooth. Pour into storage container and refrigerate.

My Timothy likes his food to taste 'sparky.' I doctored this recipe up by doubling several of the flavorings until it finally satisfied his taste buds. Experiment with it yourself!

Tomato Soup

1	can [32 oz.] **tomato** juice
½	cup raw cashew pieces
2	Tbsp. each onion powder and honey
1	tsp. sweet basil
¼	tsp. each: salt and oregano

In a saucepan, put the tomato juice (minus 1 cup). In a blender, put the cup of tomato juice and all the rest of the ingredients. Blend thoroughly (at least a minute or two) and pour into the tomato juice in saucepan and stir constantly while you heat it up.

Have only five minutes? That's about all it takes for this soup to be hot and ready to serve. We think of 'cheez' spread being served on slices of bread and broiled for 5 minutes or so with this soup. It's scrump-deliumptious!

SALSA

4	**tomatoes**
2	onions
3	green chilies
	handful fresh cilantro (if you have it available)
1	heaping Tbsp. chopped garlic
	salt to taste
1	jalapeno, seeded (optional)

In a salsa maker (if you are fortunate to own one!) or food processor put all these ingredients and work to salsa consistency. Refrigerate.

When we moved to Northern New York, Timothy saw a restaurant with the caption 'South of the Border Cuisine.' He was ecstatic—Mexican food in the north country! He was cruelly brought down however, when he was informed that there is a difference between living in New York and S. California when one reads such a line. Truly, my guy loves Mexican food, and we are still on our journey to find the ultimate homemade salsa. This is the most recent variation.

Summer Squash Medley

1	onion, chopped
4	cloves garlic, minced
1–2	Tbsp. olive oil and water
2	slender **yellow summer squash**, quartered small wedges
2	slender **zucchini**, quartered small wedges
1	can [15 oz.] tomato sauce
2	Tbsp. sweet basil
2	tsp. garlic salt
1	tsp. Italian seasoning
½	tsp. thyme

In a frying pan, sauté onions and garlic in olive oil and water. Mix all the rest of the ingredients together with this. Spoon into casserole dish, cover with foil and bake in 325° oven for 45 minutes. Just before serving, remove foil and put grated soy mozzarella cheese on top, if you want.

Note: add a small can of mushroom stems and pieces for variety.

This recipe is a user friendly one to me; especially when I am trying to use zucchini from the garden BEFORE they evolve into clones of baseball bats!

Cream of Potato Soup

8	cups water
6	large **potatoes**, peeled and cut in pieces
1	large onion, chopped
1	cup raw cashew pieces
1	cup water
2	tsp. salt
2	tsp. chicken style seasoning
¼	tsp. each: celery salt, and paprika
2	Tbsp. parsley flakes

In a saucepan, cook potatoes and onion in water until soft. Mash up potatoes with potato masher. In a blender, blend cashews and water, and all seasonings (except parsley). Add blender mixture to saucepan along with parsley. Mix all together and heat thoroughly.

The first time I made this soup, I took it to one of our homeschool get-togethers. Come lunchtime I never even got a bite—it had been totally scraped out! The next time I tried it was with a group of teenagers that were visiting our church, and the same thing happened. Neither group eats vegan, and they both loved it.

Potato Salad

6	cooked red **potatoes**, cubed
15	black olives, sliced
½	cup sweet pickle relish
¼	cup bacon-like bits
	mayonnaise

Mix all ingredients (except mayonnaise). Mix in enough mayonnaise to moisten thoroughly.

Note: you might need to adjust the amounts of relish and bacon-like bits to your liking.

This potato salad originally started out as a hot version; however, we like it just as well (or better) cold. This dish has always been a favorite when I take it to potlucks and dinners, even among non-vegetarians. I would suggest that you use red potatoes—somehow they taste the best.

Cheez Potatoes

3	**potatoes**, peeled
1	carrot, peeled

1½–2	cups water (can be the cooking liquid)
½	cup nutritional yeast flakes
½	cup vegetable oil
2	Tbsp. chicken style seasoning
1	tsp. each: salt and onion powder
½	tsp. garlic powder

In a saucepan, cook the potatoes and carrots in water until soft (can poke a knife easily into them). In a blender, blend all ingredients thoroughly. Add additional water only to keep blender going and scrape down the sides.

Scrub, peel, and partially cook 8–10 potatoes and put through the large shredder on your food processor. Mix potatoes with the cheez sauce just made and bake in 325° oven for 45–60 minutes.

This was like striking a gold mine to me when I first tasted this 'cheez.' It's great as a sauce, but we most often use it as 'cheez potatoes.' My Timothy especially likes it with lots of crust—sometimes he gets more than he bargained for when I don't hear the timer!

Hash Browns

1   **potato** *per serving (peeled if you prefer)*
½   *onion per serving*
    garlic salt to taste
    olive oil

Scrub potatoes very clean (if leaving the skins on doesn't bother you!) and put through the large shredder of food processor. Put immediately in cold water and let sit for 30 minutes. Put onions through shredder also. Oil baking sheet with olive oil. Mix potatoes and onions together and place on baking sheet and bake in 450° oven for 15 minutes; turn potatoes over and bake an additional 10–15 minutes more until golden and tender. Shake garlic salt over them and serve immediately.

I love hash browns for breakfast. If you do too and want to 'make them from scratch' this is a great way to do it.

SCALLOPED POTATOES

8	**potatoes**, peeled and thinly sliced
2	onions, peeled and thinly sliced
4	cups water
1	cup raw cashew pieces
2	Tbsp. cornstarch
1	Tbsp. chicken style seasoning
2	tsp. salt

Put the potatoes and onions in water while preparing the liquid portion. In a blender, blend ingredients from second section with 2 cups of the water until smooth. Then add the other 2 cups of water and blend again. In a casserole dish, layer potatoes and onions until all used up (I like to end with potatoes). Pour blender mixture over it all until it barely covers the potatoes (try to leave a minimum of 1 inch at top of casserole dish). Cover with foil and bake in 325° oven for 30 minutes. Remove foil and bake an additional 15–20 minutes.

Our friend Sam, from church, grows potatoes commercially. One year he gave us 5 bags (these were 50# bags!) of this wonderful vegetable! We were very motivated to find ALL recipes that used this blessing as an ingredient!

Meal-In-A-Peel

(Baked Potatoes)

1   russet baking **potato** per person scrubbed clean

      potato cheez
      sloppy joe mixture
      steamed chopped broccoli
      sour cream

Wrap potatoes in foil and bake in 325° oven for approximately 45 minutes. Heat up toppings in pretty serving dishes.

I first saw this catchy name on a menu and quickly adopted it for home. It's fun, fast, and so versatile for everyone's preferences AND a great way to use up those 2 cup portions of leftovers! (Oops! That word is on Timothy's blacklist!).

COLESLAW

½ head **cabbage**
2 carrots
mayonnaise
honey
dash of lemon juice (fresh or bottled)

Using a food processor, shred cabbage on coarse setting and carrots on fine setting. Toss together and mix with mayonnaise and a little bit of honey and lemon juice, enough to lightly cover it all. Chill before serving.

I have heard so many positive reports about 'cabbage combating cancer'! Our refrigerator houses a head of this anti-cancer vegetable year round.

Potato Salad and Sweet Beans (p. 43) ➤
Picture Perfect for a Picnic.

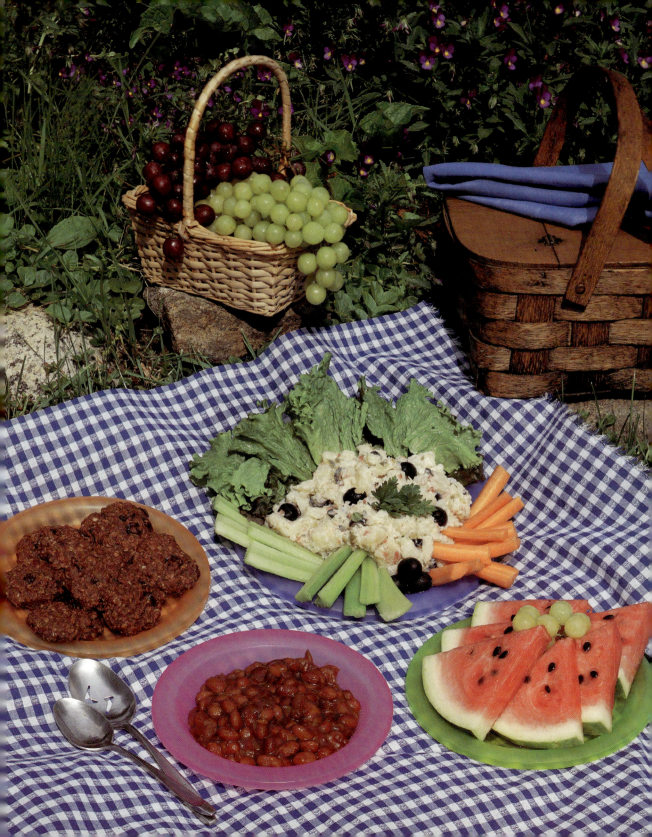

Cabbage Rolls

12	**cabbage** leaves
1	onion, finely chopped
1	garlic clove, minced
1	Tbsp. vegetable oil
1	Tbsp. water
½	cup water
1	carrot, finely shredded
1	celery stalk, finely diced
1	cup TVP
3	cups cooked brown rice
2	Tbsp. Bragg's Liquid Aminos
1	can [15 oz.] tomato sauce

Cut out core and steam cabbage leaves for 3 minutes. In a frying pan, sauté onion and garlic in oil and the 1 Tbsp. water. Add carrot, celery, TVP, and ½ cup water and continue sautéing. Then add rice and Bragg's Liquid Aminos and mix thoroughly.

To assemble put ⅓ cup portion of filling in middle of cabbage leaf, fold up (like a diaper) and place seam side down in baking dish. Pour tomato sauce over them and bake in 325° oven for 60 minutes. One option is to add 1 Tbsp. soy mozzarella jack cheese to each cabbage roll when assembling.

Note: You can freeze the head of cabbage overnight and avoid the steaming of the cabbage leaves. Once thawed, they are limp and pliable.

We were NOT cabbage roll advocates until this recipe came along. My friend Dottie regularly does cooking schools in her community and says that this recipe is ALWAYS a winner!

Glazed Beets

2	cups cooked **beets**
½	cup red cabbage, shredded
½	onion, thinly sliced
¾	cup apple juice
3	Tbsp. Sucanat®
1	Tbsp. each: cornstarch and lemon juice
½	tsp. salt

In a saucepan, mix apple juice, Sucanat®, cornstarch, lemon juice and salt. Heat over medium high heat until thickened. Add cabbage and onion and cook until they are limp. Add the beets last and heat until all is hot.

Beets find a spot in our garden each summer. They manage to do well despite our many long distance trips resulting in neglect and consequently the weeds trying to take over.

BORSCHT

4	cups julienne-sliced cooked **beets**
1	can [46 oz.] tomato juice
⅓	head green cabbage, shredded
2	Tbsp. lemon juice
½	Tbsp. onion powder

In a saucepan, put all ingredients and heat up over medium high heat until cabbage is limp. Serve hot with a scoop of 'sour cream.'

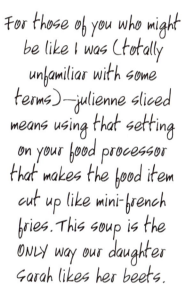

For those of you who might be like I was (totally unfamiliar with some terms)—julienne sliced means using that setting on your food processor that makes the food item cut up like mini-french fries. This soup is the ONLY way our daughter Sarah likes her beets.

Tamale Pie

½	cup TVP (rehydrated in ½ cup hot water)
½	onion, chopped
1	cup whole grain **cornmeal**
2	cups cold water
1	can [16 oz.] or 2 cups whole kernel **corn**, drained
¼	cup vegetable oil
1	tsp. salt
½	cup black olives, sliced
2	green chilies, chopped
	vegetable oil

In a frying pan, sauté TVP (mixed with the ½ cup water beforehand) and onion in small amount of vegetable oil. Mix the cornmeal with the cold water and add to frying pan mixture. After it thickens slightly, add all the rest of the ingredients and mix thoroughly. Spoon into casserole dish, cover and bake in 325° oven for 60 minutes.

We enjoy sweet corn very much during the summer and routinely can and freeze a lot of it. It's so good just plain (with salt), but sometimes we like to eat it this way. This is my variation of a recipe given to me by my friend Pauline.

Corn Chowder

2   cups whole kernel sweet **corn**
1   can [15 oz.] creamed **corn**
1   onion, finely chopped
2   cups cooked potatoes, cubed

dairy-free milk
salt to taste

In a saucepan, mix the first section together. Then add enough dairy-free milk to make a soup consistency you prefer. Heat over medium heat and add salt to taste and serve hot.

My Dad was a great cook—he grew up in a baker's family, and at an early age started pulling his share of the family's responsibilities in the kitchen. He loved making (and eating!) this corn chowder, and so I grew up eating it as a regular item on our Friday night menu—this is my variation on his recipe.

Sunshine (Carrots) Loaf

3	cups shredded raw **carrots**
2	cups cooked brown rice
2	cups bread crumbs
1	onion, chopped fine
½	cup natural peanut butter
1½	Tbsp. onion powder
1	tsp. salt
½	tsp. sage

In a large mixing bowl, mix all ingredients together. Put in a casserole dish and bake in 325° oven for 30–35 minutes.

Note: If you use peanut butter that has added oil and/or is homogenized, it will change the taste and texture somewhat.

When my friend Pattie taste-tested this recipe, her comment was, "What a delightful surprise—it tasted just like my turkey stuffing! She is not vegetarian and somewhat of a hesitant taster.

Butterscotch Pudding

3	cups cooked **carrots** (about 5 medium carrots)
2½	cups dairy-free milk
1	cup maple syrup
½	cup cornstarch
¼	cup Sucanat®
1	Tbsp. vanilla
1	tsp. maple extract
¾	tsp. salt

In a blender, blend all the ingredients (add more milk if necessary to blend). Pour into a saucepan, heat up and stir constantly until it thickens. Serve warm or pour into individual dishes and cool for a dessert dish.

Note: make sure your carrots are sweet to start with. We have found that the ones from California are always sweet.

This recipe is a fun one to try out on unsuspecting guests. They can hardly believe it's carrots! It makes a great pie, also!

Winter Squash

Blue Hubbard Squash
Acorn Squash
Butternut Squash
Turban Squash
Banana Squash

I tried for a number of years to cut squashes open with a knife and then peel the skin off the pieces any way I could. It took hours (which I don't have a lot of). My friend Joelle showed (and told) me this speedy express way of getting them from garden to oven.

Take the whole squash and throw it down on a cement slab (a sidewalk for instance). This usually breaks the squash into many pieces. Remove seeds with a sturdy spoon and wash each piece. Put pieces on baking sheets, skin side down, cover with foil and put in 350° oven for 1–2 hours. After they've cooled down, use the spoon to scoop out the fleshy food and put in a bowl. I usually add a little maple syrup and salt, mix it altogether and then freeze it in 6 cup portions (we have 6 in our family at present).

Note: these squashes will keep for a considerable length of time IF kept in cold, dark, dry storage.

Note: the seeds can be washed and roasted dry or with a little olive oil.

Pumpkin Pie

1½	cups dairy-free milk
⅔	cup roasted cashew pieces
1	cup dates, chopped
⅓	cup cornstarch
½	cup maple syrup
2	tsp. vanilla
2	tsp. coriander (can replace 1 tsp. with cardamon)
½	tsp. each: salt and orange peel
1	can [29 oz.] **pumpkin** puree

In a blender, blend the cashews with 1 cup of the milk until very smooth. Add the rest of the milk, dates, maple syrup, cornstarch, and flavorings. Pour into a mixing bowl, add the pumpkin puree and mix completely (may need to use electric beater). Put into unbaked pie shell and bake in 325° oven for 60 minutes. Let cool before slicing.

Ever since I can remember, I always wanted pumpkin pie (instead of a cake) for my birthday. Since I made the switch to vegan, I have gone through lots of recipes to find the ultimate pumpkin pie taste again. This recipe is a medley of them all...to satisfy my tastebuds.

Chunky Green Salad

Equal parts:
green peppers, *diced*
celery, *diced*
cucumbers, *sliced and quartered*
green onions, *sliced*
dried minced garlic *(optional)*

In a salad bowl, mix all ingredients. Chill and serve with your favorite creamy dressing.

While a hearty salad is essential to a healthy diet, one might not prefer leaf lettuce everyday. This salad offers the same results with a unique, delicious crunch.

Chlorophyll Salad

Equal parts:
spinach *leaves*
endive *leaves*
romaine *leaves*
iceberg lettuce *leaves*
alfalfa *sprouts*
parsley *sprigs*

Wash and rinse all leaves. CUT off any obtrusive stems or ribs that might not go well in the salad. I like to tear the pieces for this rather than cut them with a knife.

Recently, I was convinced our family needed to have more chlorophyll in our diet. Not long after, we visited my cousin Jann's home, and she served us a salad full of dark green vegetation. Phillip whispered quietly, "It looks like grass clippings!" However, I was hooked—I immediately started serving salads as full of dark-green vegetables that I could procure!

Summer Garden Salad

Equal parts:
cherry tomatoes, *halved*
broccoli, *small florets*
cauliflower, *small florets*
carrots, *thin circles*
yellow summer squash, *small wedges*
zucchini, *small wedges*

Toss together all of the above.

This salad is served in the deli section at one of the grocery stores we frequent. It is so beautiful and colorful to look at, AND it is so nutritious and delicious! If you are fortunate to be able to pick the produce right from the garden when it is young and tender, it is even more satisfying.

Minestrone Soup

4	cups chicken style broth (4 cups water: 2 Tbsp. chicken style seasoning)
1	cup **carrots**, (approximately 2 carrots) thinly sliced
½	cup each: **onions** and **celery**, chopped
1	cup medium pasta, uncooked
1	cup Italian style **green beans**
1	can [15 oz.] kidney beans, rinsed and drained
1	can [28 oz.] chopped **tomatoes**
2	tsp. Italian seasoning
1	tsp. each: salt, oregano, and sweet basil

In a large saucepan, mix all ingredients and bring to a boil. Reduce heat and simmer for 20–25 minutes.

Note: you can substitute pearl barley for the pasta.

This is a very satisfying soup. It is so filling and tastes so good.

Stuffed Peppers

3–5 **green peppers** (depends on size)

Stuffing:
1   onion, finely chopped
1   cup celery, diced
2   cloves garlic, minced
    vegetable oil

2   cups cooked brown rice
1   cup tomatoes, chopped
1   tsp. each: sweet basil, oregano, salt

melty cheese

Cut peppers in half, length-wise. Take out seeds.

In a frying pan, sauté onions, celery, and garlic in vegetable oil.

In a mixing bowl, mix rice, vegetables and seasonings. Spoon mixture into pepper halves and place in casserole dish. Spoon melty cheese on top of each one. Cover and bake in 325° oven for approximately 45 minutes.

Timothy really likes stuffed peppers and I had never had them before marrying him. So... I had to find a recipe that would satisfy us both.

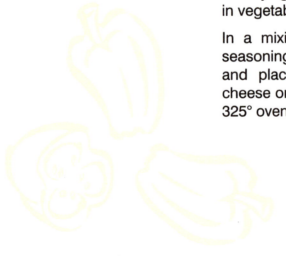

GRAINS RECIPES

Definition: the seeds of grasses

INSTRUCTIONS:

1. In saucepan put the recommended amount of hot water and ½ tsp. of salt.
2. Bring the water to a boil.
3. Add the recommended amount of grain.
4. Reduce the heat to low, cover and let cook the recommended amount of time.

COOKING GRAINS CHART

One Cup Dry Grain: **Hot Water**   **Cooking Time**

(Yields 2½ cups cooked grain)

Whole Kernels:
- barley* . . . . 3 cups . . . . 1 hour
- brown rice . . . . 3 cups . . . . 1 hour
- buckwheat groats* . . . . 3 cups . . . . 1 hour
- millet . . . . 4 cups . . . . 1 hour
- rye berries* . . . . 3 cups . . . . 6 hours
- whole wheat kernels* . . . . 3 cups . . . . 6 hours

Cracked Kernels:
- cracked wheat . . . . 3 cups . . . . 40 minutes
- cracked rye . . . . 3 cups . . . . 40 minutes
- steel cut oats . . . . 3 cups . . . . 40 minutes

Cereal Flakes:
- regular rolled oats . . . . 2 cups . . . . 15 minutes
- rolled wheat . . . . 2 cups . . . . 15 minutes
- barley flakes . . . . 2 cups . . . . 15 minutes
- rice flakes . . . . 2 cups . . . . 15 minutes
- rye flakes . . . . 2 cups . . . . 15 minutes

Coarse Meal:
- cornmeal . . . . 4 cups . . . . 10 minutes
- coarse Graham flour . . . . 4 cups . . . . 10 minutes
  (makes great Cream of Wheat!)
- whole grain Cream of Rice** . . . . 4 cups . . . . 10 minutes

*   Soak overnight prior to cooking

**   To make this: blend 1 cup brown rice to a coarse meal consistency in a dry blender. Other grains such as barley can also be done this way to make creamy quick-cooking cereals.

Bulgur Bake

2	cups **bulgur wheat**
4	cups water
½	tsp. salt
2	cups [16 oz. can] cooked garbanzos
1	onion, chopped and sautéed
1	can [8 oz.] water chestnuts
4	Tbsp. Bragg's Liquid Aminos
1	Tbsp. chives

In a saucepan, bring water to a boil. Add bulgur wheat and salt. Remove from heat and let stand for 15 minutes (or until all the water is absorbed). Let this mixture cool.

In a mixing bowl, mix cooked bulgur wheat and all the rest of the ingredients. Put into a casserole dish and bake in 325° oven for 30 minutes.

This casserole is somewhat of a plain-Jane dish. However, I wanted to include it because it does taste good and is a great way to tank up on those complex carbohydrates.

Vegeburgers with Banana Fruit Shake (p.68) for fast food atmosphere to wind down with. ➤

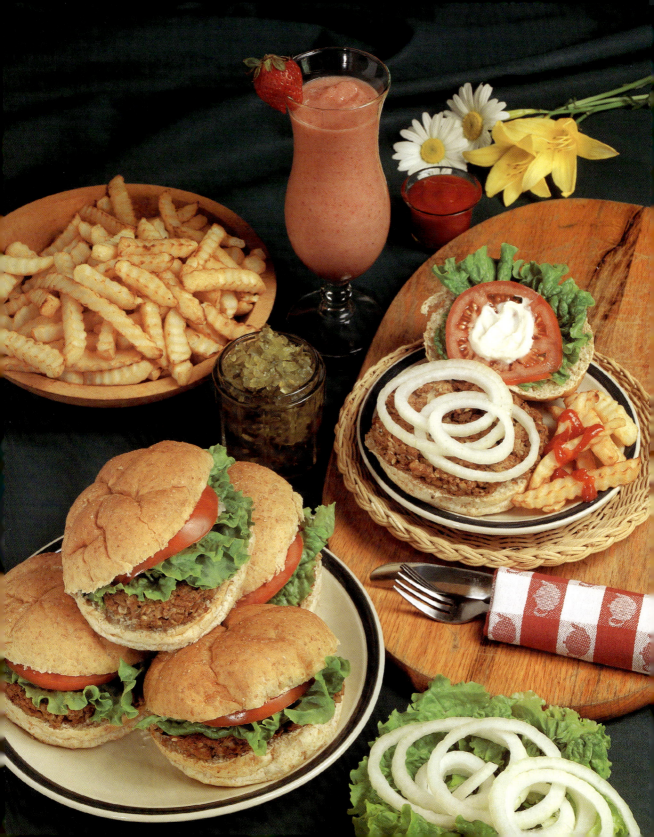

Tabouli

1	cup **bulgur wheat**
2	cups water
½	tsp. salt

1	green pepper, diced
1	cucumber, diced
2	firm tomatoes, diced

In a saucepan, bring water to boil. Add bulgur wheat and salt. Remove from heat and let stand for 15 minutes (or until all the water is absorbed). Let this mixture cool. Toss green pepper, cucumber, and tomatoes with the cooled bulgur wheat.

Make a dressing of:

4	Tbsp. lemon juice
3	Tbsp. olive oil
1	tsp. onion powder
¼	tsp. salt

Add this to the salad and serve chilled.

It wasn't until after being introduced to vegan recipes that I even knew bulgur wheat existed. It cooks up quickly and is very filling and satisfying.

SPICED RICE

2	cups dairy-free milk
4	Tbsp. cornstarch
4	cups cooked **brown rice**, cooled
2	Tbsp. honey
2	tsp. vanilla
½	cup each: shredded coconut and chopped pecans
½	tsp. each: orange peel, coriander (or cardamon)

In a mixing bowl, mix milk and cornstarch together. Then, add the rest of the ingredients and mix well. Put this in a casserole dish, cover with foil and bake in 325° oven for approximately 45 minutes.

Timothy remembers eating cooked rice for breakfast as a kid. Since he likes a lot of 'spark' to his food, I dolled up the plain-Jane rice version so it's to his liking.

Fried Rice

1	pkg. [1 lb.] tofu that's been frozen, thawed, and torn in small pieces
1	onion, chopped
	Bragg's Liquid Aminos and vegetable oil
4	cups cooked **brown rice**
½	cup green peas, frozen
	garlic salt to taste

In a frying pan, sauté tofu and onion in oil and Bragg's Liquid Aminos. Add rice and green peas. Mix thoroughly and sauté on very low heat for 20 minutes. Season with garlic salt to taste.

Note: add mushroom pieces, if you like. This is also better the second day.

The Chinese restaurant, Yonge Gardens, was our place of choice to eat as a kid growing up in Toronto. We always ordered the same thing—mushroom fried rice, chop suey, chow mein, egg foo yong, and sweet and sour soo nippets. Although I don't think we'll ever be able to match the flavor of the food, surroundings, and service of Yonge Gardens, we like this homemade version of the rice dish.

Vegeburgers

6	cups water
½	cup Bragg's Liquid Aminos
⅓	cup olive oil
4	cups regular rolled **oats**
2	cups fresh grated potato
2	cups bread crumbs
¼	cup nutritional yeast flakes
1	Tbsp. sweet basil
1	tsp. each: garlic powder and sage
1	cup walnuts, finely chopped
1	onion, finely chopped

There are lots of variations on this burger theme, and I have tried a lot of them! We HAD settled on a burger recipe, that our family really liked for years...until recently. I helped out in the kitchen at camp and came across one that we like even better. This recipe we have now crowned as the king of burgers...until a better one comes along.

In a large saucepan, combine water, Bragg's Liquid Aminos and olive oil and bring to a boil. Add oats and cook for 5 minutes, stirring occasionally. Remove from heat, add all the rest of the ingredients and mix thoroughly. Set aside for ½ hour or so to cool. Using ¼ cup portions, form patties on oiled cookie sheet and bake in 325° oven for approximately 45 minutes.

Note: this recipe makes a LOT of burgers, (approximately three dozen). We freeze in meal portions for future use.

GRANOLA

8	cups regular rolled **oats**
1	cup shredded coconut
½	cup chopped nuts (walnuts, almonds, cashews, peanuts OR pecans)
½	cup sunflower seeds
¼	cup sesame seeds

½	cup water
½	cup vegetable oil*
½	cup Sucanat®**
1	Tbsp. vanilla
½	Tbsp. each: salt and coriander

1	cup carob chips

In a LARGE mixing bowl, mix the first section (dry ingredients).

In a blender, blend the second section (wet ingredients. Pour this mixture over the dry ingredients and mix together until everything is evenly coated. Divide between 2 cookie sheets and put in oven overnight on warm OR bake in 150° oven for 2 hours, stirring occasionally. Add carob chips AFTER it has cooled. Store in airtight container.

Note: watch this carefully as it bakes, so it does not burn around the edges.

* applesauce
** chopped dates

While working at a health institute, I fell in love with a granola that one of the staff made for her family. Years later, I started making it for my family. One day not long after, I threw some trailmix into the batch I was making. It had carob chips, and it was a hit with my husband. Now granola isn't complete without the carob chips.

Delicious Millet

4 cups cooked **millet**
½ cup dairy-free milk
10 dates, chopped
½ cup shredded coconut

In a mixing bowl, mix all ingredients. Put this in a casserole dish and bake in 325° oven for approximately 60 minutes.

Note: I make this dish after the cooked millet has cooled.

"It's for the birds!" That's what my husband said when he was first served this for breakfast, a few days after our wedding. He just couldn't eat what he considered 'bird seed.' However, it wasn't too many months before this was one of his favorite dishes.

Birdseed Bread

3	cups water
1	Tbsp. salt
1	cup **millet**
1	cup regular rolled oats
1	cup flax seed
½	cup warm water
2	Tbsp. baking yeast
½	cup raw wheatgerm
⅓	cup molasses
¼	cup honey
4	Tbsp. vegetable oil
2	Tbsp. gluten flour
5–6	cups whole wheat/unbleached white

In a saucepan put water and salt and bring to a boil. Add the millet, rolled oats, and flax seed and simmer for 15 minutes. Remove from heat and set where it can cool quickly. In a 2 cup measuring cup, put warm water and yeast and set aside for 10 minutes (or until it's bubbled up). When grain mixture is at room temperature, add yeast and all other ingredients plus half the flour and mix vigorously. Add additional flour one cup at a time until it is manageable. Let rise 90 minutes. Punch down; form loaves; let rise the second time. Bake in 325° oven for 20 minutes, turn down heat to 300° and bake an additional 20 minutes (or until it sounds hollow to tapping).

I got this recipe from my friend Christin, whose husband gives it as a gift to real estate clients. It is a very sticky & seedy dough! My daughter Sarah made a loaf, hollowed it out like a birdhouse, decorated it, and gave it to her 'secret sister' from church. This bread is as edible for humans as it is for the birds!

Cornbread

2½ cups very warm water
1½ Tbsp. baking yeast
¼ cup honey

2 cups whole grain **cornmeal**
1 cup whole wheat flour
½ cup unbleached white flour
1½ tsp. salt

⅓ cup each: vegetable oil and Sucanat®

In a quart measuring cup, dissolve the yeast and honey in the water for 10–15 minutes or until it is bubbled up. In a mixing bowl, mix all the dry ingredients together. Then put in the yeast mixture, oil and Sucanat® and mix just enough to moisten. Put into baking dish (9 x 9) and let it rise in a warm place for 30 minutes. Then bake in 325° oven for about 30 minutes (or until it shows cracks on the top).

Note: this recipe will not rise much and it will be more cake-like in texture.

Cornbread reminds me of the restaurant, Marie Callendars, in S. California—where warm cornbread with honey butter is a much ordered item on the menu. My sister-in-law, Nancy, treats herself to an inside piece whenever she's visiting out there. What a treat it is!

BASIC BREAD

6	cups very warm water
½	cup honey
4	Tbsp. baking yeast
⅔	cup vegetable oil
⅓	cup molasses
2	Tbsp. salt
2	cups regular rolled **oats**
1	cup **soy** flour
1	cup **rye** flour
½	cup gluten flour
6	cups whole wheat/unbleached white

In a large mixing bowl, put water, honey and yeast and let dissolve 10–15 minutes. Then add oil, molasses, salt, oats, soy and rye, gluten flour and about 3 cups of whole wheat/white flours. Mix vigorously for about 5 minutes. Add remaining flour one cup at a time and mix until it is no longer too sticky. Take it out and knead it briefly to form a lump. Place in bowl and cover with towel. Let rise 1–1½ hours.

Punch down and form into loaves and let rise another 30 minutes. Preheat the oven to 325° and then bake the loaves for 20 minutes. Turn the heat down to 300° and continue baking for another 20–30 minutes (I normally rotate the loaves before this last 20 minutes). Take out of oven and let set for 10 minutes in pans. Then, remove from pans and place on the cooling racks.

Note: I use my Bosch mixer to make this bread. You dump everything in (in order given here), with the exception of ½ the flour. Then let it run for 5–10 minutes and add 1 cup flour at a time until the sides of the bowl come clean.

This bread is known among my family and friends as 'wonder bread'—they wonder what's in it! I've found you can add up to two cups of leftover fruit desserts, cereal, juice, or any sweet mixture, and it actually enhances the bread. My Dad told me that out of every batch of bread you make, ALWAYS give one away. I follow his advice, and enjoy the opportunity to get others hooked on whole grain goodness.

Sweet Rolls

Dough:
- 2 cups very warm water
- 1 Tbsp. baking yeast
- 1 tsp. honey

- 1 cup mashed potatoes
- ½ cup raw wheat germ
- ¼ cup dairy-free milk powder
- ¼ cup honey
- 2 tsp. salt
- 2 cups whole wheat flour
- 3 unbleached white flour

Filling:
- date butter (hot dates blended with hot water—paste consistency)
- pecan pieces, chopped
- shredded coconut
- maple syrup

In a mixing bowl, dissolve yeast and honey in water for 10 minutes. Add all other ingredients except flour. Then add flour one cup at a time, mixing in thoroughly. Knead for 10–15 minutes (use as little flour as possible). Let rise in oiled bowl for 1–2 hours.

Divide bread dough into 4 sections. With a rolling pin, roll out one section at a time in a rectangle to about 1/2 inch thickness. Spread with date butter, sprinkle with pecan pieces and shredded coconut. Roll up like a jelly roll and cut off 2 inch sections. Place in greased glass baking dish barely touching each other. Drizzle maple syrup over the top. Let rise 30 minutes. Bake in 325° oven for approximately 45 minutes.

Our family loves this breakfast menu, especially Timothy. He is very distraught if much time elapses between the times we have them. His favorite line then is "What are Sweet Rolls?" We like our sweet rolls covered with milk, and topped with sweet cream.

Flour Tortillas

2 cups **whole wheat** flour
2 cups unbleached white flour
1 tsp. salt

⅓ cup vegetable oil
1½ cups hot water

In a mixing bowl, mix all dry ingredients together; then mix in vegetable oil and hot water. It should make a floppy dough. With cutter, cut off golf ball-size pieces and roll out on a well-floured surface to a very thin circle, turning them as frequently as necessary. Cook on a dry hot frying pan for approximately a minute on each side. (You turn them over when they begin to puff up or get little bubble-like pouches in the dough).

Note: fill with refried beans, chopped veggies, salsa, olives, and cheez.

This recipe has literally traveled around the world. When my cousin Cindy was introduced to this home version recipe for flour tortillas, she liked it so much that she took it back to Africa with her. There she shared it with all the other missionaries.

BISCUITS

7½	cups whole wheat/unbleached white
2	cups quick **oats**
½	cup gluten flour
¾	cup Sucanat®
2	Tbsp. baking yeast
1	Tbsp. salt
4	cups warm water
1	cup vegetable oil

In a large mixing bowl, mix the first section (dry ingredients) together. Make a well in the middle and add water and vegetable oil. Mix with a wooden spoon until mixed enough to dump onto a floured surface. Add additional whole wheat flour (if necessary) while kneading and only knead long enough to make a workable (**NOT** stiff, but floppy) dough. With a rolling pin, roll to a thickness of 1 inch. Using a biscuit cutter, cut out the biscuits and place on oiled cookie sheet to rise for 20 minutes. Bake in 300° oven for approximately 30 minutes until lightly browned. Remove to cooling racks to cool.

Note: we freeze the extras. After they have thawed, pop them into the microwave for a minute or so and they will be soft…and of course, yummy.

Biscuits provide the foundation for our Strawberry Shortcake. We also smother them under 'Chip Beef' gravy on Monday mornings. What a wonderful way to start the week!

Soup Crackers

2 cups quick **oats**
1 cup very hot water
½ tsp. salt

2 cups **whole wheat** flour
½ cup vegetable oil

In a mixing bowl, mix rolled oats and salt with the hot water. Then add the whole wheat flour and vegetable oil and mix well. Using ½ of the dough at a time, roll between 2 pieces of wax paper until ¼ inch thick. Remove wax paper and place on cookie sheet and score (make lines with a knife where you want them to break after baking). Bake in 300° oven for 20–30 minutes until browned.

Sweet Crackers: To dry ingredients, add:

1 cup finely chopped soft date pieces
1 cup finely chopped walnuts
⅓ cup shredded coconut
⅓ cup Sucanat®

Savory Crackers: To dry ingredients, add:

½ cup onions, finely chopped
1 tsp. sweet basil
¼ tsp. garlic powder

When I first made this recipe, I was a little unsure of myself since I had always bought my crackers from the store. My kids loved them—especially the sweet crackers. They ate up the first batch before the day was out.

PANCAKES

2	cups hot water
1	cup quick **oats**
1	cup whole wheat flour
¼	cup raw cashews
1	Tbsp. Sucanat®
1	Tbsp. vanilla
½	tsp. salt

In blender, blend all ingredients at high speed for approximately 2 minutes until perfectly smooth. On a hot griddle, put ⅛–¼ cup portions per pancake. Using a spoon, smooth out rather thin. Let cook until the moisture on the up-side disappears. Turn over with a spatula and brown on the other side.

Note: these pancakes are kind of crepe-like in consistency.

Finding both a healthy and tasty pancake recipe was quite a challenge. Most I tried either fell apart or stuck so hard to the pan that I gave them up for frisbees. I usually make them 'dollar-size' and they are best hot off the griddle.

Waffles

- 2½ cups dairy-free milk
- 1½ cups regular rolled **oats**
- 1 cup whole wheat flour
- ½ cup soaked soybeans
- 4 Tbsp. vegetable oil
- 2 Tbsp. Sucanat®
- 1 tsp. salt

In a blender, blend all ingredients until smooth. Using 1 cup of batter, pour evenly onto sprayed (Pam or equivalent) hot waffle iron. Let them bake for 8–10 minutes (or according to the light indicator that is on the waffle iron).

Note: I normally make these the day ahead and then reheat them in the toaster.

Note: you may substitute soaked garbanzos or raw cashew pieces for the soybeans.

Note: you may need to add water if it is too thick.

It's a great feeling to wake up to that wonderful waffle smell tantalizing your appetite. We shared some with our friend Sam who after eating them gave his vote of confidence. Believe me, he's not one to say what he doesn't believe!

Pizza Dough

- ¾ cup very warm water
- 1 Tbsp. baking yeast
- 1 tsp. honey

- 2 cups whole wheat/unbleached white
- 1 Tbsp. vegetable oil
- ½ tsp. salt
- ¼ cup additional water (if needed)

In a medium mixing bowl, dissolve yeast in water and honey for 8–10 minutes. Add all the rest of the ingredients and mix well. On round, oiled pizza pan put dough in middle and place plastic wrap on top. Mold it all out to the edges. Remove plastic wrap. Preheat oven to 425°. Bake for 8–10 minutes. Add favorite toppings and then bake again (at a lower heat—300°) until heated through and veggies are cooked.

This is the greatest home pizza dough recipe I've found. You can make this recipe and have one "thick and chewy" OR two "thin and crispy" pizza crusts. They can be made ahead and frozen.

Pizza (p.80) toppings galore for everyone's preference ▷ Strawberry Shortcake (p.20) for dessert.

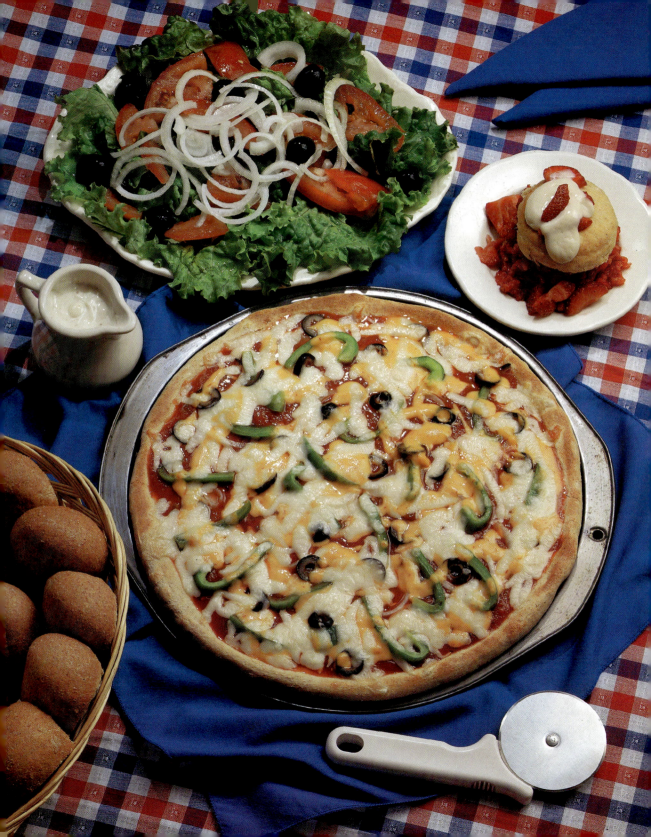

Pie Crusts

Rolled Pie Crust:

1	cup **whole wheat** pastry flour
½	cup unbleached white flour
½	tsp. salt
⅓	cup vegetable oil, cold
⅓	cup water, cold
1	Tbsp. maple syrup (optional)

In a mixing bowl, mix flours and salt together. Cut in the oil, add water and maple syrup last. It's a moist dough, and I roll it out between two pieces of wax paper. Wet the counter surface first—it'll be easier to roll.

Granola Crumb Crust:

3	cups granola (without carob chips and dried fruit)
2	tsp. coriander (or cardamon)
3	Tbsp. each: water and vegetable oil

In a blender, blend granola to a crumb texture. Remove to a mixing bowl and add the coriander, oil and water. Press into baking dish and bake 8 minutes or longer in a 325° oven. Then it will be ready for the filling.

> *I routinely use the rolled pie crust for fruit pies and the granola crust for cheesecake and the like.*

Breakfast Muffins

1½   cups **whole wheat** pastry flour
1½   cups unbleached white flour
2   Tbsp. ENER-G Foods baking powder

1½   cups warm water
½   cup apple juice concentrate
½   cup honey
4   Tbsp. vegetable oil
1   tsp. each: salt and vanilla

In a medium mixing bowl, mix the first section (dry ingredients) together. In a blender, blend the second section. Pour into the dry ingredients and mix quickly. Spoon into muffin tins ⅔ full and bake in 325° oven for approximately 30 minutes.

Note: you may substitute 2 cups of pineapple juice or apple juice for the 1½ cups water and ½ cup apple juice concentrate.

I've tried many vegan muffin recipes that I found to be more like hockey pucks than like fluffy bites of goodness. This one is hearty and ummm good... especially with fruit soup.

Bran Muffins

1	cup **wheat bran**
1	cup whole wheat pastry flour
½	cup unbleached white flour
1	Tbsp. ENER-G Foods baking powder
½	tsp. each: salt and coriander

1	cup dairy-free milk
½	cup each: barley malt and honey
4	Tbsp. vegetable oil
1	tsp. vanilla

1	cup raisins (optional)

In a mixing bowl, mix first section (dry ingredients). In a quart measuring cup (or bowl) mix second section (wet ingredients). Add wet to dry ingredients and mix just enough to moisten. Stir in raisins. Fill muffin tins ⅔ full. Bake in preheated 325° oven for approximately 20 minutes.

Thea, my friend from Emmaus Abbey down the road, shared a 20 lb. bag of wheat bran with me. Besides just adding it to foods to get additional fiber, bran muffins are a great way to eat it. This is a variation of one of Thea's bran muffin recipes. She brought me several.

Couscous Salad

2	cups water
1	cup **couscous**
½	tsp. salt
2	green peppers, diced
1	cucumber, diced (seeded if necessary)
⅓	cup fresh cilantro or parsley

Dressing:

3	Tbsp. olive oil
3	Tbsp. lemon juice
1	tsp. cumin
½	tsp. paprika
3	garlic cloves, minced

In a saucepan, bring the water and salt to a boil. Add couscous, cover and remove from heat. Set it aside for 10 minutes. Transfer to a mixing bowl, fluff with fork and let it cool completely. Add fresh veggies and the dressing. Decorate with cherry tomato halves.

When I first tasted couscous, I certainly wasn't impressed. But like flour, tofu and many other products, it needs to be seasoned and dressed up. My friend Barbara buys couscous by the 10 lb. bag and finds all kinds of interesting ways to use it. This is my variation of one of her recipes.

BEAN RECIPES

Definition: The dry seeds that are harvested from pods that grow from flowers. Also referred to as legumes.

INSTRUCTIONS:

1. Sort beans to remove any sticks, stones, or off-color beans; then wash them well.
2. Soak overnight or use the following quick soak method: In an appropriate sized saucepan put the recommended amount of water and beans and bring to a boil. Then turn off heat and cover tightly. Allow them to soak for one hour.
3. Bring beans to a boil and then cover. (If foaming is a problem, add a drop or two of vegetable oil.) Reduce heat and simmer until tender (see chart below).
4. For dry beans, peas, or lentils, teaspoon of salt for one cup of dry legumes will suit the average taste. It is best to add the salt after the beans are tender, otherwise the cooking time will be increased.
5. Alternative methods: Pressure cooking beans is the fastest way of cooking them (especially for soybeans and garbanzos). Check with your pressure cooker manual. Beans can be frozen after cooking, and this makes them readily available for any recipe you want. They can also be cooked in the crock pot overnight or baked in the oven, covered at 300° F. for 6–8 hours.

COOKING BEANS CHART

One Cup Dry Beans: *(after soaking)*	Hot Water	Cooking Time
Small Beans:		
split peas*	2½ cups	30–40 minutes
lentils, green or brown*	2½ cups	30–45 minutes
Medium Beans:		
black-eyed peas	2½ cups	30 minutes
Great Northern beans	3½ cups	½–2 hours
navy beans	3½ cups	½–3 hours
soybeans	3½ cups	12–32 hours
Large Beans:		
garbanzos	4½ cups	15 minutes
kidney beans	3½ cups	15 minutes
large limas	3½ cups	15 minutes
pinto beans	3½ cups	15 minutes

* Do not require soaking.

Most dried legumes are abundantly available. They win a gold medal for economy, flavor, ease of preparation and nutritional quality in combination with other foods. Canned legumes are available and are more convenient, but at the expense of higher cost and higher salt content.

"Chicken" Rice Soup

4	cups water
1	cup cooked **garbanzos** (or chopped chicken salad)
1	cup cooked brown rice
1	onion, chopped
2	Tbsp. chicken-style seasoning
2	Tbsp. nutritional yeast flakes
1	Tbsp. vegetable oil
	salt to taste

In a saucepan, mix all ingredients together. Cook over medium high heat until onions are transparent.

This is another one of those recipes that can come together quickly and yet taste so special—that is, if you've brought your kids up to enjoy chick-peas! My brood would rather pick them out and line them up like defeated soldiers on their plates. If you have the same problem, substitute the chicken-salad pieces from the opposite page.

"Chicken" Salad

2	cups soaked **garbanzos**
	enough water to cover in blender
¼	cup chicken-style seasoning
¼	cup Bragg's Liquid Aminos
1	Tbsp. onion powder
½	tsp. garlic powder
2	cups gluten flour

In a blender, blend soaked garbanzos (with enough water to barely cover them in the blender), chicken-style seasoning, Bragg's Liquid Aminos, onion powder, and garlic powder. Blend this mixture until smooth. Using a rubber spatula, scrape this mixture into a mixing bowl and add the gluten flour (add or subtract flour as needed to make a semi-stiff dough). Work the gluten flour in (it will NOT act like bread dough!) until you can form it into a flattened lump that you can put on a greased cookie sheet. Bake this in 325° oven for approximately 60 minutes or until it is brown. Remove to a cooling rack and let it set until completely cooled off. Cut into pieces that you can put through a food processor on a coarse blade. Freeze in 2 cup portions.

Note: to make sandwiches, add mayonnaise and chopped celery and/or onions and put on rye bread.

I have yet to find a reluctant taster that hasn't been pleasantly surprised with this salad. One of my friend's sons doesn't profess any health interest, and will eat practically anything that crawls across his plate. After the first bite of this in a sandwich, he was hooked.

Chick Pea Salad

2	cups cooked **garbanzos**
8	cherry tomatoes, halved
½	cup green onions, chopped
½	cup fresh basil
2	cloves fresh garlic, minced

Dressing:

1	Tbsp. each: olive oil and lemon juice
1	Tbsp. each: sweet basil and parsley
	dash paprika and salt

In a salad bowl, mix garbanzos and veggies. Mix seasonings with liquid, shake well and toss in with salad.

A main salad to go along with any meal to satisfy hungry appetites.

Great Gravy

2	Tbsp. Bragg's Liquid Aminos
1	Tbsp. vegetable oil
1	onion, finely chopped
2	cups water
1	cup cooked **garbanzos**
⅓	cup whole wheat flour
¼	tsp. each: celery salt, garlic powder, and salt

In a frying pan, sauté onion in oil and Bragg's Liquid Aminos. In a blender, blend garbanzos in 1 cup of the water until smooth. Add other cup of water and all other ingredients and blend again. Pour into frying pan with onion and stir with whisk until thickened.

A good gravy to add to the meal-in-a-peel options.

Three Bean Salad

1	cup [15 oz. can] cooked **garbanzos**
1	cup [15 oz. can] cooked **kidney beans**
1	cup [15 oz. can] cooked cut green beans
10	black olives, sliced
2	green olives, sliced
2	onions, sliced

Dressing:

2	Tbsp. each: olive oil, lemon juice, honey, and Bragg's Liquid Aminos.

Combine with the bean mixture. Refrigerate overnight and serve chilled.

In a mixing bowl, mix beans and veggies.

This dish was one of Timothy's favorites at the deli section when he used to eat out all the time. Now, in a homestyle version, it is still just as satisfying as any restaurant could offer.

Black Beans

4	cups cooked **black beans**
2	onions, chopped
2	green peppers, diced
2	cloves garlic, minced
3	Tbsp. vegetable oil
3	Tbsp. lemon juice

In a saucepan, mix all ingredients together. Add enough water to make it soup-like. Bake for 1 hour in 325° oven.

As a newlywed, I was trying my best to impress Timothy with both unique and delicious-looking dishes. I'll never forget the first time I served him these black beans; he absolutely refused to eat them. He agreed that they were unique—they were the wrong color! Not long ago, he purchased a couple of cases of black beans—quite the change from a man who wouldn't even try them!

Savory Soybeans

4	cups cooked **soybeans**
2	cups canned tomatoes (or tomato sauce)
½	cup Sucanat®
1	can [6 oz.] tomato paste
¼	cup lemon juice
1	Tbsp. dried parsley
1	tsp. each: salt and sweet basil
1	onion, chopped
	vegetable oil

In a frying pan, sauté onions in a small amount of water and vegetable oil. Then in a casserole dish mix all ingredients together. Bake for one hour in 325° oven.

Years ago, our family was given many pounds of soybeans. At the time (with very young children), there wasn't enough time to spend on making recipes like soy milk, tofu, etc. from scratch. I decided to experiment in making a bean dish with them. We like this one.

Esau's Pottage

1	onion, chopped
2	Tbsp. vegetable oil
4	cups cooked **lentils**
½	cup cooked brown rice
1	can [6 oz.] tomato paste
2	carrots, diced
1	Tbsp. dried parsley
1½	tsp. each: sweet basil and onion powder
1	tsp. salt

In a saucepan, sauté onion in a small amount of vegetable oil. Mix together all ingredients. Heat thoroughly over medium high heat.

I can see how Esau fell for such a pot of lentils. I first had this dish at my Aunt Betty's house and fell in love with the taste. Beforehand, lentils were not a favorite! It is most tasty served with warm whole wheat bread on a cold winter day.

Navy Bean Soup

3	cups cooked **navy beans**
5	cups water
2	cups potatoes, cubed
2	cups fresh/frozen kale
2	Tbsp. nutritional yeast flakes
1½	tsp. salt
¼	tsp. cumin
1	onion, chopped
2	garlic cloves, minced
2	Tbsp. olive oil

In a frying pan, sauté onions and garlic in olive oil. In a large saucepan, put this with all the rest of the ingredients and cook over medium high heat about 20 minutes. Serve immediately.

My friend Patty spent a number of years in Africa where there was an abundance of greens to eat with their meals. This recipe sounded kind of weird to me until she served it to me. I had been so accustomed to eating navy beans as sweet beans; so this savory dish is a delightful diversion.

Sweet Beans

4	cups cooked **navy beans**
1	cup dates, chopped
½	can [6 oz.] tomato paste
½	cup dried onions
¼	cup molasses
2	tsp. salt

In a casserole dish mix all ingredients. Bake for one hour in 325° oven.

Note: If I'm in a hurry, I substitute ½ cup Sucanat® for the dates.

Sweet Beans have to be one of my all-time favorites. It was a dish my Mom made many Sabbaths for lunch. One of my close friends likes to tease me about eating particular dishes only with another certain dish. I have to admit that Sweet Beans wouldn't be what they are without its counterpart, Potato Salad.

ENCHILADAS

1   pkg. [12] corn tortillas
1   pkg. Soya Kaas mozzarella cheese
6   green chilies
1   can [15 oz.] vegetarian **refried beans**
1   can [15 oz.] tomato sauce
1   pkg. [1¼ oz.] Taco seasoning
    olive oil

Brush one side of corn tortillas with olive oil. Microwave (all stacked on top of each other) for approximately 1–2 minutes. Mix tomato sauce with seasoning. Cut cheese in half. Make 12 strips of one half and shred the other half.

To assemble one tortilla, spread with 1 Tbsp. tomato sauce, put one strip cheese, one 'strip' of beans, and ½ chile. Fold over both sides and place seam side down in casserole dish. Do all 12 (2 rows of 6 each). Drizzle remaining tomato sauce on top and shred remaining cheese on top. Bake in 325° oven for 1 hour.

Timothy has always loved Mexican Food. I make these up ahead so when I have to be away he can relish his lunch; otherwise it's granola and canned peaches when I'm gone.

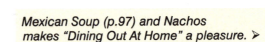

Mexican Soup (p.97) and Nachos makes "Dining Out At Home" a pleasure. ➤

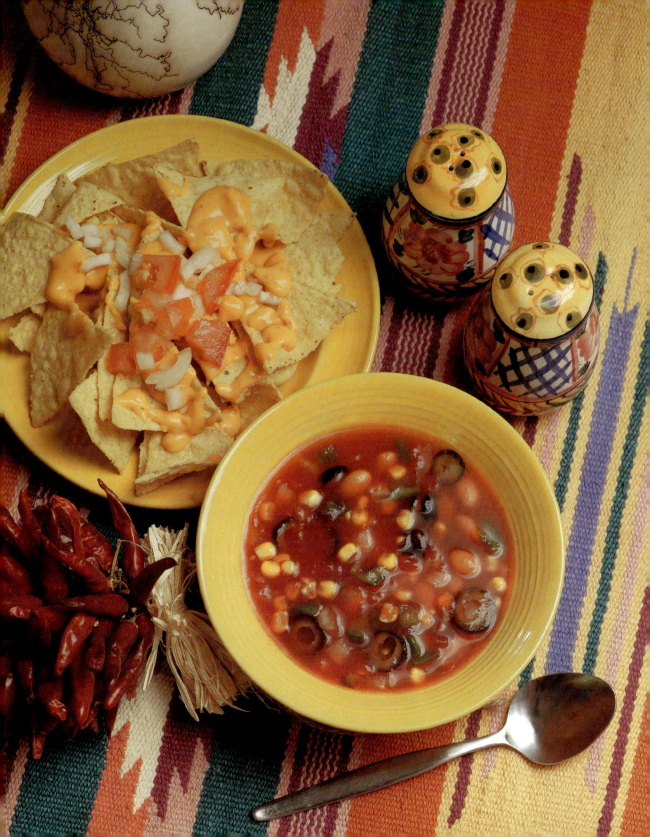

Mexican Soup

2	cups cooked **pinto beans**
4	cups canned tomatoes (blended slightly)
2	cups whole kernel corn
1	onion, chopped
1	green pepper, diced
½	cup black olives, sliced
½	tsp. cumin
¼	tsp. garlic powder
½	pkg. [1¼ oz.] Taco Seasoning
1	small can green chiles (optional)

In a large saucepan, mix everything all together and cook over medium high heat until vegetables are tender, about 30 minutes.

A bowl of soup is an easy meal to get for a group of people without much hassle. Our home-schooling group will often each bring a part of this recipe, throw it all together in a huge pot and let it cook while we do our activity.

Split Pea Soup

2 cups dry **split peas**
6 cups hot water
1 onion, chopped
1½ tsp. each: salt and onion powder
¾ tsp. sweet basil
¼ tsp. garlic powder

dairy-free milk
bacon-like bits

In a saucepan, soak the split peas in the hot water for 60 minutes. Add onion, salt, onion powder, sweet basil and garlic powder, Cook this over medium high heat until the split peas are soft and mushy (approximately 60 minutes). In a blender, blend about 2 cups of this mixture at a time until creamy smooth. Add dairy-free milk as you are blending to get the right consistency. Serve hot with bacon-like bits as a garnish.

Elwozetti, a South African friend of mine, was initially having a hard time adjusting to the differences in our cultures, particularly dietary. She tasted this soup, loved it and saw brighter horizons ahead.

Sloppy Joes

	vegetable oil
1	cup vegetarian burger (or TVP)
1	onion, chopped
2	cups cooked **kidney beans**
1	cup spaghetti sauce

In a frying pan, sauté vegetarian burger/TVP and onion in a small amount of vegetable oil. Add kidney beans and spaghetti sauce. Heat thoroughly and serve over whole wheat buns.

Sloppy Joes sure live up to their name. Besides being sloppy, they are also very good to eat. They are very good over any kind of bread, but our family likes to use it for our 'meal-in-a-peel' option, also.

CHILI

4	cups cooked **pinto beans**
2	cups stewed tomatoes
1	onion, chopped
2	Tbsp. each: molasses and lemon juice
1	Tbsp. chili-like seasoning
2	tsp. sweet basil
1	tsp. salt
¼	cup bulgur wheat or vegeburger

In a saucepan, mix all ingredients together and cook over medium heat for approximately one hour.

Chili and cornbread or chips are inseparable in our home. Because there are two kinds of "hot" (temperature & spice) I have to make sure it is served only during winter—which is not too hard here in the north country—we only get two months of 'summer.'

NUTS & SEEDS RECIPES

Definition: a hard-shelled dry fruit or seed with a separable rind or shell and interior kernel.

Almonds – a small tree of the rose family.

Cashews – a tropical American tree with small kidney shaped fruit.

Coconut – a large seed from the coconut palm. Each nut contains white meat with a milky liquid.

Peanuts – not a true nut, but rather a legume (bean). Grows underground.

Pecans – a large hickory from Central and Southern United States with thin shells.

Sesame Seeds – an east Indian plant whose seeds are most commonly used on buns or ground to make tahini.

Sunflower Seeds – a large flower with the appearance of the sun.

Walnuts – a large shade tree also used for lumber. These nuts are the most common nut used in cooking.

Coconut Cream Frosting

¼ cup raw **almonds**, blanched (skins removed)
1 cup cold water
1 Tbsp. maple syrup
dash salt

1 cup Sucanat®
4 Tbsp. cornstarch
¼ cup water

½ cup shredded coconut
1 cup pecans, chopped

In a blender, blend almonds, water, maple syrup, and salt until very smooth. Pour into saucepan and add Sucanat®, cornstarch, and water. Stirring constantly, cook over medium high heat until thickened. Add coconut and pecans and spoon over cake. Let cool.

This frosting is good over the carob prune cake.

Coconut Cream Pie

- 2 cups [13.5 oz. can] coconut milk
- 1 cup water
- 1½ cups raw cashew pieces
- 1 cup corn syrup
- ¼ cup cornstarch
- 1 Tbsp. vanilla
- ½ tsp. salt

- ½ cup shredded **coconut**

In a blender, blend all ingredients (except coconut). In a saucepan, heat blender mixture, stirring constantly until thickened. Spoon into prebaked pie crust, sprinkle coconut on top and chill.

This recipe is actually the fallout from a banana cream pie recipe. Timothy said, "Blah! I like the texture, but the taste leaves a lot to be desired." So we experimented and this is what we came up with.

Coconut Macaroons

2	cups shredded **coconut**
½	cup whole wheat flour
½	tsp. salt
½	cup honey
¼	cup dairy-free milk
1	tsp. vanilla

In a mixing bowl, mix the first section (dry ingredients) together and then add the second section (wet ingredients). Form teaspoon-size cookies on oiled cookie sheet and bake in 300° oven for 20 minutes.

Note: they don't hold together real well when you form them on the cookie sheet, but they stick together real well after they are baked and have cooled down.

My Dad loved macaroons, and as a kid I never even thought of trying to make them from scratch for him. But I try to do everything that way now, and so this cookie is no exception.

Maple Pecan Cookies

3	cups quick oats
½	cup whole wheat flour
½	cup unbleached white flour
½	cup **pecans**, chopped
½	cup shredded coconut
½	cup Sucanat®
1	tsp. salt

½	cup maple syrup
½	cup vegetable oil
1	tsp. vanilla
½	tsp. maple flavoring

In a mixing bowl, mix first section (dry ingredients) together. Make a well and add second section (wet ingredients). Mix all together and drop by teaspoonfuls on cookie sheets and bake in 325° oven for approximately 15–20 minutes.

I love maple syrup and these cookies certainly are enhanced with its flavor. I knew they were user-friendly when my friend Richard asked for the recipe.

Nut Butter Cookies

Many vegan cookie recipes I've tried are stiff, dry and somewhat on the bland side. This cookie recipe erases this memory.

½ cup natural peanut **butter or almond butter** (smooth or crunchy)

¼ cup each: honey and vegetable oil

⅓ cup tahini

1 tsp. vanilla

½ cup whole wheat pastry flour

¼ cup unbleached white flour

½ cup Sucanat®

½ tsp. salt

In mixing bowl, cream together first section (wet ingredients). Then add last section (dry ingredients) and mix thoroughly. Form small balls of dough, place on cookie sheet and flatten with fork to a thickness of approximately ½ inch. Bake in 325° oven for 12 to 15 minutes. Do not let them get very brown. Remove from sheets when cooled.

Note: you can substitute applesauce for the oil.

Seed Samplers

3   cups assorted **seeds** (sesame, sunflower, pumpkin, flax)
½   cup each: barley malt and honey

In a small saucepan put barley malt and honey. Heat up, stirring constantly, until boiling. Remove from heat and mix in seeds. Spoon small mounds onto greased cookie sheet. Let cool.

Note: Add ½ cup carob chips to sweeteners for a different flavor.

Not long ago, I started peddling my seed supplements to the family. While it didn't bother me to gulp down a handful of seeds, the kids were appalled by the idea. So I had to come up with another strategy. I bought some sesame seed chews as a snack item for my health food store. My kids liked them so much, I decided to make a similar item myself.

French Toast

1½	cups water
1	cup quick oats
⅓	cup raw **cashew** pieces
2	Tbsp. vegetable oil
2	Tbsp. Sucanat® (or honey)
1	tsp. vanilla
½	tsp. salt

whole wheat bread slices

In a blender, blend all ingredients until smooth. Pour into shallow bowl and coat slices of whole wheat bread on both sides. Let drip a second or two, and then place on oiled cookie sheet. Bake in 325° oven for 10 minutes. With a spatula, turn them over and bake an additional 10 minutes.

French toast is one of my favorite dishes, and is very easy to make when it is baked. This is, of course, much healthier!

"Chip Beef" Gravy

3	cups hot water
1	cup raw **cashew** pieces
4	Tbsp. cornstarch
4	Tbsp. vegetable oil
2	Tbsp. Bragg's Liquid Aminos
4	tsp. onion powder
1	tsp. salt
½	tsp. garlic powder
½	cup bacon-like bits

In a blender, blend all ingredients (except bacon-like bits) until very smooth. Pour into saucepan, rinse out blender with one additional cup of water and pour that also into the saucepan. Add bacon-like bits and cook over medium high heat, stirring constantly until thickened. Serve over biscuits.

Note: this will scorch if not watched carefully.

This is traditionally our Monday morning breakfast and one that our whole family looks forward to. No leftovers at this meal!

Veggie Dip

½	cup **tahini**
1	pkg. [12.3 oz.] firm silken tofu
4	Tbsp. vegetable oil
2	Tbsp. lemon juice
1	Tbsp. honey
1	tsp. each: salt and dill weed
½	tsp. each: onion and garlic powder
¼	cup each: black olives, red and green peppers and onions, finely chopped

In a blender, blend all ingredients (except olives and veggies) until very smooth. Add olives and veggies. Refrigerate.

Tahini is a seed spread made from ground-up sesame seeds. It has been my experience that folks either love it or leave it. This dip is very smooth and filling.

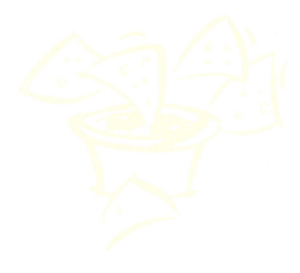

Sour Cream

1	cup boiling water
⅔	cup raw cashews
½	cup **sunflower seeds**
⅓	cup lemon juice
½	tsp. each: salt and onion powder
¼	tsp. garlic powder

In a blender, blend all ingredients until very smooth. Refrigerate.

When I think of sour cream, baked potatoes or borscht comes to mind. When I found this recipe it had the basic look and texture I wanted.

I made it several times, experimenting with various quantities of the seasonings, and this is the end result.

Pecan Roast

1	onion, chopped
2	stalks celery chopped
	vegetable oil
1½	cups **pecans**, finely chopped
3	cups bread crumbs
2	cups dairy-free milk
¾	cup regular rolled oats
¼	tsp. sage

In a frying pan, sauté onions and celery in the vegetable oil. In a mixing bowl, mix all ingredients together. Spoon into casserole dish and bake uncovered in 325° oven for 30–40 minutes.

When I first made this roast, my kids turned up their noses at it. Finally, after getting them to taste it, they now agree that not all casseroles are that bad.

Lasagna (p.115) with a side dish of broccoli, it's a mouth watering response. ➤

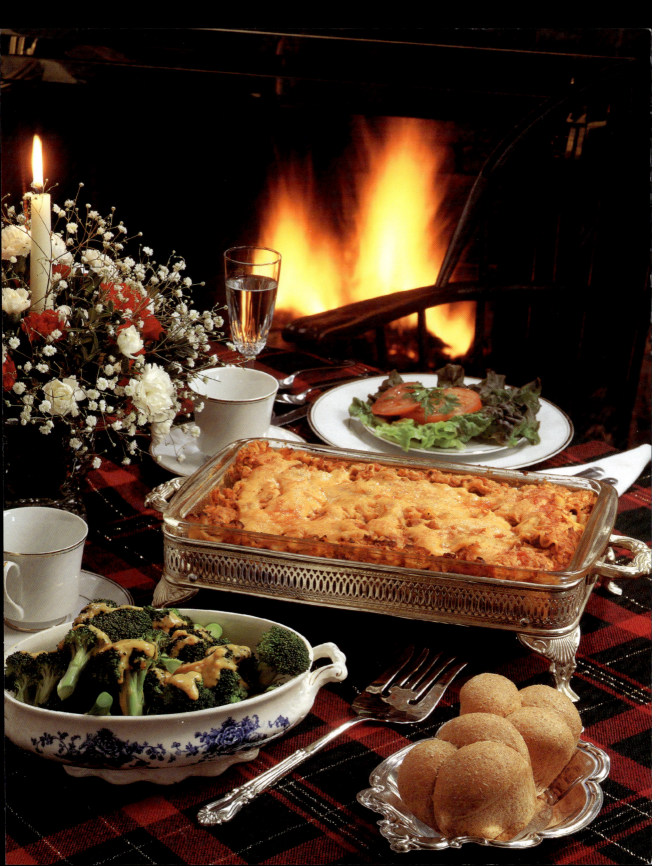

MISCELLANEOUS

The main ingredients for the recipes in this section you won't find growing on any tree or picked in any garden. They are set here because they have a specific nutrient/ratio that is not as the original food.

Macaroni and "Cheese"

8	cups water
1	tsp. salt
4	cups **macaroni shells**
1	cup "cheese"

In a saucepan, bring water and salt to a boil Add macaroni shells and stir. Lower heat to medium high and cook 8–10 minutes or until tender. Drain.

Mix cooked macaroni with cheese. Add more cheese if you want. Bake in 325° oven for approximately 60 minutes, until crusty on top.

Sarah makes this for Friday lunch, every chance she gets. Whenever we are away on long trips, this is the meal we all most long for. I usually set out salsa to top it with.

Lasagna

8–12 cups water
1 tsp. salt

9 **lasagna noodles**

spaghetti sauce
crumbled tofu
"cheese"

In a saucepan, bring water and salt to a boil. Drop in the lasagna noodles and cook 8–10 minutes. Drain. Mix the tofu with the cheese (so it resembles cottage cheese).

Layer the following spaghetti sauce, cooked lasagna noodles, tofu/cheese mixture. Repeat. Finish with tomato sauce. Drizzle plain cheese sauce over the top. Bake in 325° oven for one hour.

Note: this dish tastes even better when reheated the next day.

This is one of our special Sabbath dishes. It was only after showing my friend Laurie how to put this recipe together, that I realized you can layer it more than just 3 sections! I sure do get in a rut at times! That's why it's good to share and receive with others.

Pasta Salad

8   cups boiling water
1   tsp. salt

4   cups dry **veggie spirals**

      mayonnaise
      black olives, chopped
      celery, diced
      pimentos, chopped
      relish

In a saucepan, bring water and salt to a boil. Add veggie spirals and cook 8–10 minutes, or until tender. Drain.

Add mayonnaise, chopped black olives, diced celery, chopped pimentos and relish. Serve chilled.

Donna, a homeschooling friend of mine, is responsible for this becoming a regular part of our dietary regime.

Spaghetti and "Meatballs"

1	onion, finely chopped
2	Tbsp. vegetable oil

1	cup TVP
1	cup bread crumbs (not toasted)
1	pkg. [12.3 oz.] silken tofu, mashed
½	cup walnuts, finely chopped
4	Tbsp. nutritional yeast flakes
2	Tbsp. cornstarch
1	tsp. each: sage and garlic powder
½	tsp. salt

In a frying pan, sauté onion in oil. Remove to mixing bowl and add all the rest of the ingredients. Form into walnut-size balls and bake in 325° oven for about 45 minutes.

Note: I make these ahead and freeze, so all you need to do is reheat them.

This is our 'instant' meal if we're very hungry and don't have much time. Again, our kids like their food very plain so don't care much for the 'meatballs' but I like them and so have included them here.

MAYONNAISE

1	pkg. [12.3 oz.] firm silken **tofu**
1/3	cup vegetable oil
1/4	cup lemon juice
1½	Tbsp. onion powder
2	tsp. salt
1/4	tsp. garlic powder

In a blender, blend all ingredients until smooth. Run the blender on high, scraping down the sides until it turns stiff and won't blend any longer. Refrigerate.

Growing up, I was brought up on Hellman's Real Mayonnaise; Timothy was brought up on Miracle Whip. Trying to combine these two tastes to make a palatable mayonnaise was challenging. This recipe has the look and texture and most of the taste we want.

SWEET CREAM

1	pkg. [12.3 oz.] of extra-firm silken **tofu**
2	Tbsp. vegetable oil
⅓	cup maple syrup
⅓	cup Sucanat®
1	tsp. vanilla
¼	tsp. salt

In a blender, blend all ingredients until very smooth. (I use a rubber spatula to scrape down the sides until all of the mixture is blended smooth.) Refrigerate.

Sweet cream is our version of 'cool-whip.' We use it as a topping on pies, crisps and cobblers. Sometimes we use it as a spread for bread. But add carob powder (approximately 2 Tbsp.) to it, and it becomes a pudding to layer with sliced bananas and topped with granola. Very delicious!

Tofu Soufflé

2	cups (16 oz. pkg.) firm tofu
¼	cup vegetable oil
2	Tbsp. each: pimentos, cornstarch, nutritional yeast flakes
1	tsp. each: salt and Bragg's Liquid Aminos
½	tsp. each: garlic powder and turmeric

In a blender, blend all ingredients until thoroughly mixed. Spoon into pie pan and bake in 325 oven for 45–60 minutes.

Note: for a quiche-like dish, blend in 1 package of frozen spinach and leave out the pimentos and turmeric. The rest of the recipe is the same.

For me, a Soufflé was always a favorite restaurant choice. This is a very tasty choice option, but not a clone.

Scrambled Tofu

2	cups [16 oz. pkg.] firm **tofu**, cubed
1	Tbsp. chicken-style seasoning
1	Tbsp. nutritional yeast flakes
2	Tbsp. vegetable oil
1	tsp. Bragg's Liquid Aminos
½	tsp. each: turmeric, onion powder and salt
2–3	garlic cloves, minced (optional)
1	Tbsp. dried onions (optional)

In a frying pan, sauté all ingredients thoroughly. Brown over medium high heat until heated through.

Our friend Alan comes up each year for 6–8 weeks to work on his pipe organ handbook. The first year he came, the thought of eating vegetarian food for 6 weeks scared him. Before arriving at our house, he went out to eat and loaded up with all his favorites, trying to tank up for the meatless drought. He has since become vegetarian, and now THIS is a favorite... about twice a week.

TOFU CHEESECAKE

1	cup frozen pineapple juice concentrate
¼	cup frozen apple juice concentrate
3	Tbsp. Emes Kosher-Jel
½	cup raw cashew pieces
⅓	cup honey
1½	pkgs. [12.3 oz.] extra firm silken **tofu**
1	cup coconut milk
2	tsp. vanilla
½	tsp. each: lemon juice and salt
1	prebaked granola crust

In a saucepan, heat up the first section, stirring constantly. In a blender, blend this mixture with the second section. Add the third section and blend again. Pour into granola crust and chill in refrigerator for at least 6 hours. Top with thickened blueberries.

The first time I tried to make a tofu cheesecake, Timothy dutifully ate a piece. When he declined to have a second piece, I knew I had to search until I found an appetizing one that warrants a second piece. This is it.

Eggless Salad

2	cups X-firm silken **tofu**, crumbled
½	cup mayonnaise
2	Tbsp. all purpose seasoning (page 129)
½	cup each: celery and onions, finely chopped

In a mixing bowl, mix the mayonnaise, seasoning and veggies. Add the crumbled tofu. Serve as a relish or in a sandwich.

My friend Dottie raved so much about the egg salad recipe she uses, that I decided to try it and we liked it. I reworked it a little which cut down on preparation time and fit my schedule better.

Gluten Steaks

3½	cups **gluten flour**
2½	cups water
1	cup soaked garbanzos
¾	cup walnuts
¾	cup regular rolled oats
½	cup nutritional yeast flakes
1	tsp. salt

While helping out with a health program years ago, I suggested this recipe be used in the menu for the Banquet Dinner. The meal was catered by chefs unfamiliar with cooking vegetarian. Imagine my surprise at the Banquet a few weeks later when set before me was this huge steak-like creation. Obviously the cooks had taken the name literally, and had made 'steaks.'

In a blender, blend all ingredients, except gluten flour. Pour into a mixing bowl and add gluten flour, one cup at a time, mixing in thoroughly with a wooden spoon and kneading when you can. Form a sausage-like roll, cover with plastic wrap and refrigerate overnight. Then cut into ½ inch slices, roll with a rolling pin on floured surface and boil in broth (recipe below) for at least 2 hours. This recipe makes a lot, so you can plan to freeze meal-size portions.

Broth:

18	cups hot water
1	cup Bragg's Liquid Aminos
3	onions, chopped
3	stalks celery, sliced
1	green pepper, chopped
4	cloves fresh garlic, minced
6	Tbsp. chicken-style seasoning
1	Tbsp. salt

In a very LARGE pot, combine all ingredients. Follow directions above.

Stroganoff

1	onion, chopped
6	**gluten steaks**
	vegetable oil
	Bragg's Liquid Aminos
1	recipe chip beef gravy (without bacon-like bits)
½	cup mayonnaise

In a frying pan, sauté onion and strips of gluten steaks in equal parts of vegetable oil and Bragg's Liquid Aminos. In a saucepan, mix gravy and mayonnaise. Add the onions and gluten to gravy, heat all together. Serve hot.

This is a special meal I enjoy very much. I serve it most of the time over brown rice with a side dish of steamed broccoli.

"Cheese"

2	cups water
⅔	cup nutritional yeast flakes
⅓	cup unbleached white flour
¼	cup vegetable oil
¼	cup canned sweet red peppers
2	Tbsp. each: cornstarch and lemon juice
2	tsp. salt
1	tsp. onion powder
¼	tsp. garlic powder

In a blender, blend all ingredients together until very smooth. Pour into saucepan and cook over medium–high heat until thickened, stirring almost constantly.

When my sister's family was visiting us, I served haystacks with this cheese. The kids were little, and quite picky. They hardly touched the chopped vegetables and the beans, but they piled this cheese on with no problem, and really liked it! We make it weekly...sometimes more.

Mustard

1	cup water
⅔	cup lemon juice
½	cup unbleached white flour
⅓	cup vegetable oil
1	Tbsp. turmeric
1	tsp. salt

In a blender, blend all ingredients until very smooth. Pour into saucepan and cook over medium heat until thickened. Refrigerate.

I was not brought up using mustard so have not felt the need to find a look-alike. However, over the years I've used this one in cooking schools and it has been well received as a clone.

Tacos

3   cups vegeburger
       (or rehydrated TVP)
1   onion, chopped
       vegetable oil and Bragg's Liquid Aminos
½   pkg. [1.25 oz.] Taco Seasoning

In a frying pan, sauté vegetarian burger/TVP, onion in small amount of vegetable oil and Bragg's Liquid Aminos. Add Taco seasoning. sauté until golden brown. Remove from heat and then build tacos.

Not long ago, Timothy brought home a case of taco shells that he "got a good deal on!" We ate tacos quite frequently! I have since added refried beans occasionally to the TVP mixture and we like it that way also.

Chip Beef Gravy (p.109) over Biscuits (p.76) ➤ for a garden brunch.

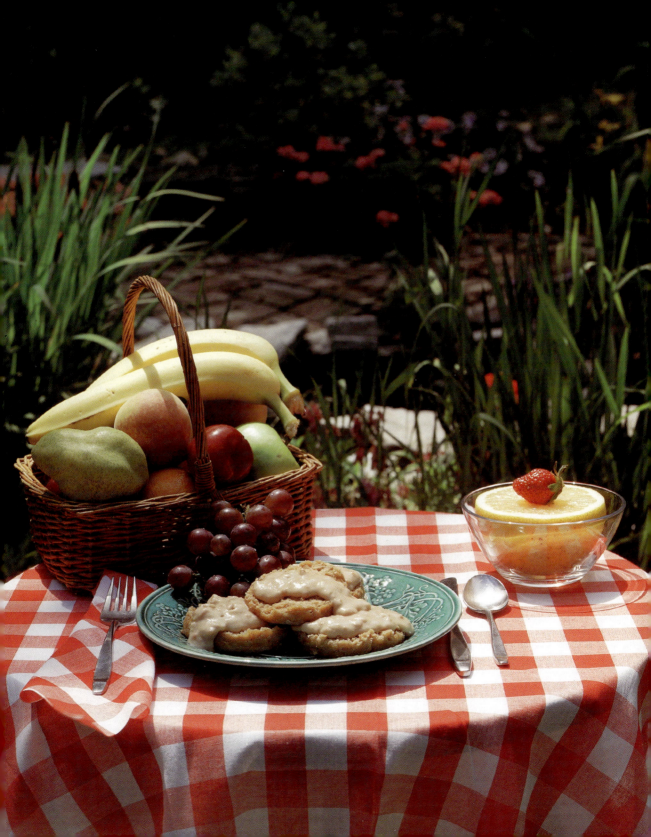

All Purpose Seasoning

- 1 cup nutritional yeast flakes
- 3 Tbsp. salt
- 1 Tbsp. each: onion powder and paprika
- 2 tsp. garlic powder
- 1 tsp. parsley
- ½ tsp. each: celery salt and turmeric

In a mixing bowl, mix all ingredients together. Store in airtight jar.

This seasoning is made up ahead of time.

Chili-Like Seasoning

2 Tbsp. each: paprika, cumin and cayenne
1 Tbsp. each: oregano and garlic powder
1 tsp. each: sage and thyme
½ tsp. turmeric

In a small mixing bowl, mix all ingredients together. Store in airtight container.

Some like it hot, some like it cold... this pre-made seasoning helps give the additional spark to dishes that my husband likes.

KID'S KORNER

This section is for all kids 5-12 years old OR those who are kids at ♥ !!

Have fun!

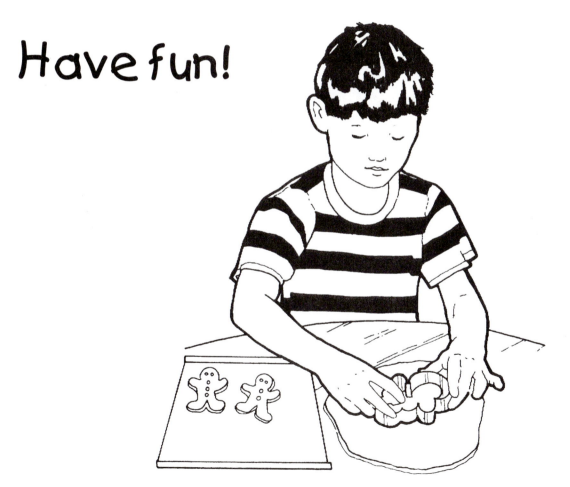

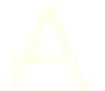

Baked Apple

yellow or red delicious apple
chopped dates/raisins/nuts
sweet cream

is for

APPLE

Core out the middle of the apple. Stuff with chopped dates or raisins and/or favorite chopped nuts. Put in a covered casserole dish and bake in 325° oven for approximately 30 minutes. Serve hot with a scoop of sweet cream.

Banana Logs

banana
creamy peanut butter
raisins
green & red grapes

is for

BANANA

Set a peeled banana on a plate. Drizzle creamy peanut butter along the top. Place a few raisins on it (these are ants!). Make 'people' with the grapes and toothpicks.

Celery Go-Carts

crisp celery
peanut butter
1/4 inch thick round peeled carrot
toothpicks

C is for CELERY

Cut celery into 2-3 inch pieces. Fill with a small amount of peanut butter. Cut slices off carrot, and with two toothpicks serving as axles, put these 'wheels' on.

Date Nut Chews

dates
honey bear
walnuts

D is for DATE

Split open date; take pit out. Squirt a small amount of honey inside date; place walnut inside and squeeze shut, put in mouth and chew and chew.

Fresh Fruit Kabobs

1. pineapple chunks
2. kiwi slices
3. whole strawberries
4. banana slice
5. green grapes

½ cantaloupe
shish kabob sticks

Put fruit on stick in order given. Turn the cantaloupe upside down on a plate and stick the colorful sticks into the cantaloupe.

Mashed Potato Volcano

hot mashed potatoes
sauce of your choice
(i.e. tomato, cheese or brown-gravy)
parsley sprigs

Mound potatoes on a plate, make a dent in top with a spoon and ladle some sauce in top. Place parsley 'trees' all over the mountain to look like a forest.

Happy Face

round waffles
peanut butter
coconut
banana
apricot
kiwi
date

Spread waffle with peanut butter. Cut banana in half and use one for the smile. Peel kiwi and cut in circles for eyes. Sprinkle coconut on top for hair. Put apricots on for ears and date for nose.

Haystacks

1. bag of corn chips
2. can of refried beans
3. iceberg lettuce, shredded
4. tomatoes, chopped
5. onions, chopped
6. olives, sliced
7. salsa
8. melty cheese
9. sour cream

Heat up the beans. Layer every ingredient in order given. Delicious!

Mud Pies

1 recipe pie crust dough

1 1/2 cups dairy-free milk
1 cup Sucanat®
6 Tbsp. each: cornstarch, carob powder and peanut butter
4 Tbsp. whole wheat flour
2 tsp. vanilla
1 tsp. coffee substitute
1/2 tsp. salt

1 cup granola

Roll out walnut-size portions of pie dough and form in small muffin tins. Bake in 325° oven for approximately 10-15 minutes until slightly brown.

In a blender, blend all ingredients in middle section until smooth. Pour into a saucepan and heat over medium high heat until thickened, stirring constantly (it scorches easily!). Remove from heat, add granola and spoon in baked pie crusts. Let cool and then enjoy!

Teddy Bear Bread

Step 1. In a measuring cup, put:
 1/2 cup warm water
 1 Tbsp. baking yeast
 1 squirt honey from honey bear
 Set aside for 5-10 minutes, until all bubbled up.

$$1/4 + 1/4 = 1/2$$

Step 2. In a bowl, mix:
 1 cup boiling water
 1/2 cup quick oats
 2 Tbsp. vegetable oil
 2 Tbsp. molasses
 1 tsp. salt
 Set aside for 5 minutes.

Step 3. Mix steps 1 & 2 together and mix real well with wooden spoon. Add 1 cup whole wheat flour and 1/2 cup unbleached white flour and knead for approximately 10 minutes. Add more flour if necessary.

Step 4. Cut dough in half. Form one half as the body. Cut the other half in half again. Take one of these halves and form the head. Cut remaining half in 7 pieces... 2 ears, 1 nose, 4 paws. Use raisins for decorations. Let rise for 30 minutes.

$$1/2 + 1/2 = 1$$

Step 5. Bake at 325° for approximately 20 minutes. Watch carefully so he doesn't burn!

Bird's Nest

3 cups rice crispies
1 cup shredded coconut

3/4 cup dairy-free milk powder
1/2 cup each: honey and peanut butter
2 Tbsp. vegetable oil
1 tsp. vanilla

In a mixing bowl, mix first section. In a saucepan, bring to a boil the second section, stirring constantly. Pour over dry mixture and mix until all is evenly cooled. Wait until it cools, so it can be handled. Form bird's nests and chill. Fill with your favorite "eggs." We like to use carob-covered peanuts.

Note: homogenized peanut butter will react differently than natural peanut butter; add more rice crispies and milk powder as needed.

Cup of Carob

2 Tbsp. carob powder
2 Tbsp. honey
1 tsp. vanilla
2 cups dairy-free milk

In a blender, blend all ingredients. Pour into mugs for you and your friends, and heat in microwave.

O.J. Jel

1 can frozen orange juice concentrate
1 can water
2 Tbsp. Emes gelatin

In a saucepan, bring all ingredients to a boil. Remove from heat and pour into bowls and refrigerate.

Snowman

½ cup each: Sucanat®, lite corn syrup and water
2 Tbsp. vegetable oil
2 tsp. vanilla

6 cups popped corn

In a saucepan, heat all ingredients except popcorn over medium high heat until it reaches 220° F on candy thermometer (approximately 3-5 minutes). Remove from heat and pour over popcorn. Stir with a spoon to coat all the popcorn. As soon as it is cool enough to handle (before it becomes brittle) form into balls and build a snowman.

INDEX

BEANS

"Chicken" Rice Soup 86
"Chicken" Salad 87
Black Beans 91
Chick Pea Salad 88
Chili 100
Enchiladas 96
Esau's Pottage 93
Great Gravy 89
Mexican Soup 97
Navy Bean Soup 94
Savory Soybeans 92
Sloppy Joes 99
Split Pea Soup 98
Sweet Beans 95
Three Bean Salad 90

FRUITS

Applesauce Toast 36
Apricot Couscous 25
Apricot Jam 24
Banana Fruit Shake 14
Banana Nut Bread 15
Berry Good Cobbler 32
Blueberry Breakfast Cake 22
Blueberry Pie 23
Carob Prune Cake 18
Cranapple Crisp 30
Cranberry Relish 31
Fruit Soup 26
Fruit/Nut Bites 27
Lemon Chiffon Pudding 17
Orange Ambrosia 28
Orange Julius 29
Peach Crisp 35
Pineapple Pudding 16
Prune Crisp 19
Rhubarb Crisp 33
Strawberry Shortcake 20
Strawberry Yogurt 21
Tropical Fruit Gel 34

GRAINS

Basic Bread 73
Birdseed Bread 71
Biscuits 76
Bran Muffins 83
Breakfast Muffins 82
Bulgur Bake 64
Cornbread 72
Couscous Salad 84
Delicious Millet 70
Flour Tortillas 75
Fried Rice 67
Granola 69
Pancakes 78
Pie Crusts 81
Pizza Dough 80
Soup Crackers 77
Spiced Rice 66
Sweet Rolls 74
Tabouli 65
Vegeburgers 68
Waffles 79

KIDS KORNER

Baked Apple 132
Banana Logs 132
Bird's Nest 138
Celery Go-Carts 133
Cup of Carob 139
Date Nut Chews 133
Fresh Fruit Kabobs 134
Happy Face 135
Haystacks 135
Mashed Potato Volcano 134

Mud Pies 136
O.J. Jel 139
Snowman 140
Teddy Bear Bread 137

MISCELLANEOUS

"Cheese" 126
All Purpose Seasoning 129
Chili-Like Seasoning 130
Eggless Salad 123
Gluten Steaks 124
Lasagna 115
Macaroni and "Cheese" 114
Mayonnaise 118
Mustard 127,129
Pasta Salad 116
Scrambled Tofu 121
Spaghetti and "Meatballs" 117
Stroganoff 125
Sweet Cream 119
Tacos 128
Tofu Cheesecake 122
Tofu Soufflé 120

NUTS AND SEEDS

"Chip Beef" Gravy 109
Coconut Cream Frosting 102
Coconut Cream Pie 103
Coconut Macaroons 104
French Toast 108

Maple Pecan Cookies 105
Nut Butter Cookies 106
Nut Roast 112
Seed Samplers 107
Sour Cream 111
Veggie Dip 110

VEGETABLES

Borsch 51
Butterscotch Pudding 55
Cabbage Rolls 49
Cheez Potato 44
Chlorophyll Salad 59
Chunky Green Salad 58
Coleslaw 48
Corn Chowder 53
Cream of Potato Soup 42
Glazed Beets 50
Hash Browns 45
Ketchup 38
Meal-In-A-Peel (Baked Potatoes) 47
Minestrone Soup 61
Potato Salad 43
Pumpkin Pie 57
Salsa 40
Scalloped Potatoes 46
Stuffed Peppers 62
Summer Garden Salad 60
Sunshine (Carrots) Loaf 54
Tamale Pie 52
Tomato Soup 39
Winter Squash 56

We would love to send you a free catalog of titles we publish
or even hear your thoughts, reactions, criticism,
about things you did or did not like about this
or any other book we publish.

Just write or call us at:

TEACH Services, Inc.
254 Donovan Road
Brushton, New York 12916-9738
1-800/367-1998

http://www.teachservicesinc.com